EMBRACING YOUR INNER CRITIC

Embracing Your

Inner Critic

Turning Self-Criticism
into a Creative Asset

Hal Stone, Ph.D. & Sidra Stone, Ph.D.

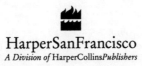

HarperSanFrancisco
A Division of HarperCollins*Publishers*

To Irene Lillian Liggett
February 6, 1892–December 20, 1991

HarperSanFrancisco and the authors, in association with the Rainforest Action Network, will facilitate the planting of two trees for every one tree used in the manufacture of this book.

FIRST EDITION

Library of Congress Cataloging-in-Publication Data
Stone, Hal.
    Embracing your inner critic: turning self-criticism into a
creative asset / Hal Stone and Sidra Stone.—1st ed.
      p. cm.
    ISBN 0-06-250757-5
    1. Criticism, Personal. 2. Self-talk. I. Stone, Sidra, 1937–.
II. Title.
BF637.C74S76 1993   92–53894
158'.1—dc20   CIP

93 94 95 96 97 ❖ CWI 10 9 8 7 6 5 4 3 2 1
This edition is printed on acid-free paper that meets the American National Standards Institute Z39.48 Standard.

CONTENTS

PART 1
Introducing Your Inner Critic

PART II
How the Inner Critic Operates

PART III
The Inner Critic and Relationship

PART IV

Transforming the Inner Critic

ONE

Introducing
Your Inner Critic

Chapter One

_____

What Is Your Inner Critic and Where Did It Come From?

On the journey of self-discovery, let us stop looking for what is wrong with us. Let us discover, instead, who we are and how we work! Let us put our judgment aside as we explore the amazing system of selves within us and learn to live with ever-increasing honesty, choice, and freedom.

There was once a dreadfully wicked hobgoblin. One day he had a simply marvelous idea. He was going to make a looking glass that would reflect everything that was good and beautiful in such a way that it would look dreadful or at least not very important. When you looked in it, you would not be able to see any of the good or the beautiful in yourself or in the world. Instead, this looking glass would reflect everything that was bad or ugly and make it look very important. The most beautiful landscapes would look like heaps of garbage, and the best people would look repulsive or would seem stupid. People's faces would be so changed that they could not be recognized, and if there was anything that a person was ashamed of or wanted to hide, you could be sure that this would be just the thing that the looking glass emphasized.

The hobgoblin set about making this looking glass, and when he was finished, he was delighted with what he had done. Anyone who looked into it could only see the bad and the ugly, and all that was good and beautiful in the world was distorted beyond recognition.

One day the hobgoblin's assistants decided to carry the looking glass up to the heavens so that even the angels would look into it and see themselves as ugly and stupid. They hoped that perhaps even God himself would look into it! But, as they reached the heavens, a great invisible force stopped them and they dropped the dreadful looking glass. And as it fell, it broke into millions of pieces.

And now came the greatest misfortune of all. Each of the pieces was hardly as large as a grain of sand, and they flew about all over the world. If anyone got a bit of glass in his eye there it stayed, and then he would see everything as ugly or distressing. Everything good would look stupid. For every tiny splinter of the glass possessed the same power that the whole glass had!

Some people got a splinter in their hearts, and that was dreadful, too, for then their hearts turned into lumps of ice and could no longer feel love.

The hobgoblin watched all this and he laughed until his sides ached. And still the tiny bits of glass flew about.

And now we will hear all about it. . . .

Adapted from "The Snow Queen,"
by Hans Christian Andersen

The Inner Critic is like the bit of mirror that makes us see a distorted picture. It is that inner voice that criticizes us and speaks about us in a disparaging way. It makes everything look ugly. Most of us are not even aware that it is a voice or a self speaking inside of us because its constant judgments have been with us since early childhood and its running critical commentary feels like a natural part of ourselves. It develops early in our lives, absorbing the judgments of the people around us and the expectations of the society in which we live. When we talk about this critical voice, please keep in mind that this Inner Critic is the voice within us that criticizes us, whereas the Judge is the self within us that criticizes other people.

THE INNER CRITIC AS A CITIZEN OF THE WORLD

As we traveled around the world and worked with people from many different cultures, we were amazed at the power and universality of the Inner Critic. It might wear a different costume, but it was easily recognizable! Whether we were teaching in Europe, Israel, Australia, or the United States or working with people from Japan, China, or Southeast Asia, we found that the Inner Critic was always present. The content of its criticisms, however, varied according to the value system of each particular culture. We have been particularly fascinated by these variations.

For example, in America your Critic is likely to criticize you if you are not special enough or if you are not superior to others. Your Critic does not want you to disappear into the crowd, to be ordinary. Australian Critics take the opposite view. In Australia they have a saying that goes something like this: "Don't be a tall poppy because tall poppies get their heads cut off." You are not supposed to stand out, to be special, or to do anything that will draw special attention to you. Holland and other northern European countries with a strong Calvinist background have a similar value structure, and there too it is important not to stand out, even if you have done something special. In these countries, the Inner Critics are quite judgmental toward people who stand out too much or who try to be special.

The great similarity we have noted among all the Inner Critics of the world is their ability to cripple people and to keep them unhappy and ineffective. Although it is interesting to think of what life would be like without this critical voice, in reality we can never get rid of it, nor would we want to. As we shall see in the course of this book, the Critic can become our ally once we learn to recognize it and to handle it. However, as long as we are unconscious of it, we must constantly appease it.

YOU CANNOT PLEASE YOUR INNER CRITIC

No matter how much you try, you cannot please your Inner Critic. No matter how much you listen to it and try to change yourself in the way that it wants, it follows you and grows stronger. It is exactly like a parent who has been critical of you. Nothing that you do is okay. It is also like a dragon that keeps growing more heads as long as you do not deal with it. The harder you try to change yourself, the stronger it gets. Try to please it, and it will grow. The answer is to learn how not to play the game, and that is what this book is about—learning not to play the critic game.

RADIO STATION KRAZY

The Inner Critic has been with us since we were small children. It was born early in our lives in an attempt to protect us and keep us safe. What is important for us to realize here is that the Inner Critic has been broadcasting like a radio station since we were small children, announcing all the things that are wrong with us. We call this station KRAZY. Since it has been broadcasting for decades, the vast majority of us no longer hear it, for it is like background music and we no longer notice that it is playing.

It often happens that when people become aware of the Inner Critic and finally begin to catch hold of station KRAZY, they will say to us, "You know, I've heard that voice all my life. I just thought it was me!" We say to you unequivocally that *the Inner Critic is not you!* It is a voice in you that has developed for specific reasons. It is not a voice that has to run your life forever!

THE INNER CRITIC HAS SUPERSTAR BILLING

As we shall see, many different selves make up our individual persons. The reason that we give the Inner Critic superstar billing is that it is the one voice in us that is able to stop our personal growth entirely, or at least to stunt it severely. It blocks our ability to live a creative life. How does this happen?

Let us say that it is midnight and you have gone to the kitchen and eaten two delicious peanut butter and jelly sandwiches. Once you have finished eating, the Inner Critic really starts to tear you down. It tells you how terrible you are, what a slob you are. It tells you that you have no self-control and never will have any self-control. It tells you that you are a blimp and that it hates you, that it is disgusted by you. The litany of your sins can go on endlessly, and soon the act of eating two peanut butter and jelly sandwiches has become a major crime against humanity.

This kind of voice stops all growth. It is almost impossible to work on the issue of food and what it means to us when this voice has made our midnight party into a crime against humanity. It makes us feel so bad about the sandwiches—it so humiliates and shames us—that the Critic itself becomes the major problem. The issue is no longer the meaning of food in our lives and how we use it and need it to handle stress and anxiety. The issue now is how to handle the attack of an out-of-control critical voice that has turned eating into a major disease. Once the Inner Critic has reached this level of authority, it is not uncommon for people to be required to eat, smoke, drink, or use drugs, sex, or exercise in a compulsive way in order to cover up the bad feelings that come from these Critic attacks. The original issue is lost and the Critic is now the problem.

Once you understand that this is the voice of your Inner Critic, that radio station KRAZY is playing, then you have choices and it is possible to begin to take greater control over this area of your life. You can learn to turn down the volume or turn off the radio. You can learn to change to another station. Eventually, you can even learn to change the nature of the programming on this station. You *can* learn to change the behavior and attitude of this Inner Critic. First, however, you must learn to hear the music.

WHERE DID YOUR INNER CRITIC COME FROM?

In considering where the Inner Critic came from, always keep in mind that *the Inner Critic's original function is to spare us shame and pain*. This will help to keep things clear as we explore the development of the Critic and its purpose in our lives. In the growing-up process your parents have to teach you to look good and to behave appropriately in order to succeed in the world, both at home and in the workplace. After all, who would be to blame if you turned out badly? So your parents look at you, try their best to figure out what is wrong with you, and then do what they can to fix it. The same is true of relatives, teachers, religious leaders, people at your workplace, and general acquaintances. Being fixed, and trying to fix others, is a major part of human interactions.

Mothers usually notice that you do not look quite right and try to correct the problems they think they see. They let you know their concerns about your looks and they discuss how to improve matters. They tell you to bathe or to wash your hair or to stand up straight in order to improve your appearance. They put you on a diet either to make you thinner or to make you fatter. They curl your hair or they straighten your hair. They tell you what is wrong with the way you dress or, perhaps, how much better someone else dresses or how much better someone else looks.

Some mothers are more indirect about the way they try to fix you, pointing out what is wrong with the way other people dress or act so that you will know what you should not do. Some mothers do not say anything. They just look at you with a worried expression and you have to guess what is wrong with you!

Your father observes that you are not careful enough when you help him with the chores or when you do your homework, so he points out what you are doing wrong or tells you that you are clumsy or careless. He wants you to be disciplined, careful, and clever. He wants you to be able to figure things out and to solve problems. As you listen to him, you begin to feel pretty stupid. Parents need to succeed in making you a proper person—whatever that means to them—in order to feel good about themselves. Underneath all this is their own insecurity and their own fear of failure as parents.

Some aspects of your behavior make your parents pretty uncomfortable. They do not like it when you interrupt them, when you are noisy, when you are angry, or when you cannot sit still. Your curiosity and your sexuality may embarrass them.

When you do not obey them, they get annoyed. When they want you to sleep, they want you to sleep whether or not you are sleepy. They want you to eat what they want you to eat, and they do not necessarily take your taste into consideration. You must eat what is good for you and at the times that are convenient for them. There are lots of things about you that your parents want to change just because they are who they are!

No matter what their motivation, the basic message you receive from your parents in all of this is: "There is something wrong with you." The implication is that if only you would improve yourself all would go well for you.

In order to protect ourselves from the pain and the shame of always being found less than we should be, a voice develops within us that echoes the concerns of our parents, our church, or of other people who were important to us in our early years. We literally develop a "self," a separate subpersonality, that criticizes us before our parents—or anyone else, for that matter—can!

The Inner Critic is a self (or subpersonality) that develops to protect us from being shamed or hurt. It is extremely anxious, almost desperate, for us to succeed in the world and to be accepted and liked by others. It is not the only self that lives within us. You can read in detail about our many selves, how they develop, and how they operate in relationships in our books, *Embracing Our Selves* and *Embracing Each Other.*

WHAT DOES THIS INNER CRITIC SOUND LIKE?

The Inner Critic is remarkable in a number of different ways. It seems to operate with heightened awareness in all areas. It can see, hear, and feel what is wrong with us as though it had the most advanced technology at its disposal. It has the intelligence of a genius, an uncanny intuition, an ability to analyze our feelings and motivations, a sweeping gaze that notices the tiniest of details, and, in general, an unerring ability to see and to magnify all our faults and shortcomings. It seems to be a lot more intelligent and perceptive than we ordinary mortals are.

If you listen carefully, you can hear it whispering in your ears at most any time. Here are some of its favorite statements:

The trouble with you is. . . .

You're basically ugly. Nothing you ever do will help.

You're not really loveable. Or, Nobody really likes you.

You're selfish.

You're mean.

You're basically flawed.

You look dreadful.

You're fat.

You're flabby.

You're too short. Nobody takes short people seriously.

You're getting old.

That outfit is all wrong. You look ridiculous.

You have no talent.

You're boring.

You shouldn't have said that.

If you didn't work twice as hard as everyone else, you'd never make it.

You need to have your nose done.

You may have fooled them into thinking you're smart, but wait until they find out the truth about how little you really know.

You are really a fake underneath it all.

These are just a few of the Inner Critic's statements. The Inner Critic uses words in powerful ways. One its favorite words is *mistake*. It dearly loves this word. "That was a mistake. I should not have gone to lunch. I should not have sent that letter. I should not have eaten that sandwich. I should have said yes to that invitation." Behind all these "should nots" and "shoulds" is the basic assumption that we erred, that we made a mistake. A mistake is unacceptable and we feel miserable whenever we think we have made one.

In looking at the Critic's use of language, we must not forget the word *symptom* and other related ways of describing things. Extra weight becomes a symptom. Having too much to eat becomes a symptom. A headache becomes a symptom. Too much coffee becomes an addiction. A strong attachment to another person becomes *addictive* behavior. The need for others, which is universal, becomes *codependency,* a new diagnostic category. It is not that there is no merit in some of these terms. They have proven very helpful to people who are combating certain kinds of behavior. The problem is that the Inner Critic picks these terms up and uses them as weapons against our growth.

Imagine that someone becomes ill and a New Age friend says to that person, "You created your illness and you are responsible for your health." Think of someone with cancer or some serious illness and just imagine what the Inner Critic does with that. Tuning in to the Inner Critic is an amazing experience as we begin to hear how powerful and all-pervasive are the judgmental voices that surround us and feed the Critic in our society.

WHAT DOES YOUR CRITIC REALLY WANT AND HOW DOES IT ACTUALLY AFFECT YOU?

The Inner Critic really wants you to be okay. It really wants you to make it in the world, to have a good job, to make enough money. It really wants you to be loved, to be successful, to be accepted, to have a family. It developed in your early years to protect your vulnerability by helping you to adapt to the world around you and to meet its requirements, whatever they might be. In order to do its job properly, it needed to curb your natural inclinations and to make you acceptable to others by criticizing and correcting your behavior before other people could criticize or reject you. In this way, it reasoned, it could earn love and protection for you as well as save you much shame and hurt.

However, the Inner Critic often does not know when to stop. It does not know when enough is enough. It has a tendency to grow until it is out of control and begins to undermine us and to do real damage. Its original intent gets lost in the sands of time. Like a well-trained CIA agent, the Inner Critic has learned how to infiltrate every portion of your life, checking you out in minute detail for weakness and imperfections. Since its main job is to protect you from being too vulnerable in the world, it must know everything about you that might be open to attack from the outside.

But, like a renegade CIA agent, at some point the Critic oversteps its bounds, takes matters into its own hands, and begins to operate on its own agenda. The information, which was originally supposed to be for your overall defense and to promote your general well-being, is now being used against you, the very person it was meant to protect. With the Critic's original aims and purposes forgotten, all that is left for it is the excitement of the chase and the wonderfully triumphant feeling of conquest, as it operates secretly and independently of any outside control.

When the Critic starts to outgrow its initial usefulness in this way, there is real trouble. At this point, the Inner Critic makes you feel dreadful about yourself. With your Inner Critic watching your every move, you become self-conscious, awkward, and ever more fearful about making a mistake. You may even stop trying because the Critic tells you that you are going about things all wrong and will undoubtedly fail. Although, underneath all of this, the Critic may want you to be so perfect that you will not fail, its effect is to block any attempts you might make.

The Inner Critic kills your creativity. How can you possibly try anything new or different when you know that you will do something wrong?

The Inner Critic, on an inner level, is the source of low self-esteem. How can you possibly feel good about yourself when you have a voice inside of you that is telling you nonstop what is wrong with you?

The Inner Critic is a source of shame. It finds every aspect of the natural "you" unsatisfactory, and it is relentlessly trying to change everything. There is no part of you that can avoid its piercing gaze—even the depths of your feelings, dreams, and impulses that you might be able to hide from the outside world.

The Inner Critic can make you depressed. If your Critic is running your life without any balance coming in from elsewhere, its constant barrage of criticism can be extremely debilitating and discouraging. This can lead to physical and psychological exhaustion and depression.

THE INNER CRITIC AND THE INNER FAMILY OF SELVES

The Inner Critic is not alone. It is only one of a number of primary selves that make up our personality and define who we are in the world.

Each of us is born into this world a unique human being. We are born with a genetic make-up that will determine our physical appearance and will, to some extent, affect our behavior. In addition to this, we are born with our own "psychic fingerprint," a unique and indefinable but clear quality that identifies us and makes us different from everyone else. It is this quality that you think of when you think of a particular person. It has nothing to do with physical appearance or behavior; it is far more subtle. This psychic fingerprint is carried by our initial self, the Vulnerable Child who will be with us throughout our lives. Last, but not least, we are born with the inherent capacity to develop any number of selves. These selves are the building blocks of the personality we will have as we grow older.

As infants, we are extremely sensitive and quite open to everything that happens around us and to us. We are totally dependent upon others for the love and the care that we need to survive. We are in a state of complete vulnerability. Without proper caretaking, we will not live to grow up.

What can we do to ensure that we survive? What can we do to be sure that others do not hurt us and that they take care of us? To meet these needs, we develop a personality that both protects us and makes us attractive to others. This personality is made up of a group of subpersonalities, or selves, that helps us to fit into our environment. These selves are called "primary selves" because they are primary in our lives—they determine who we are and how we act.

As we develop these primary selves, we move away from our initial psychic fingerprint and we adapt to the world around us. Imagine an infant in the crib. It wants to feel good, to be smiled at, picked up, and hugged. There is someone, a mother, looking down at it. The infant discovers that when it smiles, this mother smiles back. She is warm and happy and she picks up the child and holds it. She makes sweet loving sounds. Life is good.

THE PLEASER

The infant, although it may truly feel like smiling much of the time, soon learns that smiling is an important act. Life is much better when it smiles. Thus, one of the earliest *primary selves* is born, the Pleaser. This Pleaser begins to override the natural tendency to smile and makes the child smile more frequently than it would ordinarily without the Pleaser's instructions. This way, the mother will be happy. This makes the infant safe and the world feels a good deal nicer. With the Pleaser as a primary self, we make others happy and they, in turn, make us happy. In this way our vulnerability is protected.

Now that the Pleaser has become a primary self, opposite energies (or selves) must be kept away so that the Pleaser can do its job properly. The infant learns that when it is unhappy or angry and it cries loudly, it will be ignored or, perhaps, spanked. At best, its mother will try to stop its crying, but she is not the same happy loving mother that responds to the Pleaser. The crying makes her tense and irritable, and the world just does not feel as good as it did when the Pleaser was in charge. So the infant learns that crying is bad and anger becomes what we call a *disowned self. The disowned self is a self that is pushed away and not allowed into our conscious lives. It is equal and opposite to the primary self that makes up our personality.* We may know that it is there underneath, but we try our best to keep it down. The infant may know that it wants to cry, but it stifles this reaction. If this continues long enough, and if the Pleaser gets strong enough, the young child may not even be aware that the anger or the tears are there at all.

This gives you a picture of the way our personalities develop. As we have said, our personalities are made up of a group of primary selves that determine who we are and how we behave. They make our decisions for us automatically. We have no choice so long as we are not aware of them. If the Pleaser is one of my primary selves, I must be nice to you and accommodate myself to your wishes, and I actually have no choice in the matter. It is not that I am being dishonest or manipulating you. It is simply that I, or actually my Pleaser, *must* put your needs before mine.

It is ironic that the Vulnerable Child, whose protection is the aim of the primary selves, gets lost in all this. We must develop a personality, a set of primary selves, to protect this Vulnerable Child or we will not survive. However, in protecting it, we bury it.

Becoming aware of these selves inside of us changes the way in which the primary selves operate in our lives. Becoming aware of the primary selves gives birth to an Aware Ego, which we will describe at the end of this chapter. This Aware Ego is then in a position to take over gently from the primary selves that have cared for us over the years and to assure them that it can keep us safe. The development of this awareness and of an Aware Ego to replace the Ego that has been operating is an extremely important aspect of Inner Child work.

THE RULE MAKER

We have talked a bit about the development of the Pleaser and the disowning of anger. Now let us show you how some of the other primary selves develop, because these all work closely with the Inner Critic. Each of us has a Rule Maker who makes up the rules about what kind of person we should be and what kinds of characteristics are unacceptable. This part of us develops early in life to protect our vulnerability. It looks around us, sees what is rewarded and what is punished, and it develops a set of rules for us to live by that will keep us safe.

For instance, if you grow up in an average middle–class American family, your Rule Maker would probably want you to be sensible, successful, hardworking, honest, dependable, an achiever, fairly well behaved, cheerful, outgoing, self-assured, attractively dressed, and neatly groomed. These qualities will be reflected in your primary selves. Your Rule Maker will probably not want you to be lazy, sloppy, angry, too sexual, too emotional, loud, inappropriate, shy, unattractive, dishonest, or selfish. These equal and opposite qualities will become your disowned selves.

Your Critic works hand in glove with this Rule Maker. It is your Critic's job to help you to live up to the standards set by your Rule Maker who, generally speaking, sounds like the voices of parents and society blended together on an inner level. Your Critic will keep a close eye on you to be sure that you do not fall below the standard that has been set. Needless to say, the standard is impossible for anyone but Superman to attain, but it is there, nonetheless. This relationship between the Inner Critic and Rule Maker is essential to understand because the Critic's job is to uphold the rules that have been established.

To learn to handle the Inner Critic means that we also must learn to separate from the Rule Maker. For instance, if the Rule Maker wants us to be competent and self-assured, the Critic will review our behavior and find any signs, either overt or covert, of incompetence or insecurity. Even if any objective observer would think that we had done a great job, our Inner Critic, knowing what was going on inside of us, is able to find the flaws in either our performance or our inner attitude.

THE PUSHER

The Pusher is another major primary self in many of us and a great teammate of the Inner Critic. It usually develops to help us do well at school. The Pusher's job is to get us to achieve, to meet goals, to keep moving forward in life. It helps us to get ahead in the world. The Pusher is never satisfied. We can always do more or do it faster or better. It sets ever-changing requirements for us. Just as we reach the goal line, wherever it may be, the Pusher runs ahead of us and moves the goal a bit farther on, so that again it is out of reach. With a strongly developed Pusher, we are like racing dogs running after an artificial rabbit that we can never catch.

Your Pusher has developed as a primary self to gain recognition for you and to assure your success in the world. In our culture, we admire the person who does the most, who sets the records. Our parents try very hard to get us to be hard workers, and it must be admitted that most of us would not accomplish much without the aid of a Pusher. But the Pushers of the world have a tendency to be a bit too ambitious.

We have noticed that New Age Pushers absolutely love bookstores. We estimate that a large percentage of books are purchased by the Pushers of the world, especially the New Age Pushers. Once we have the books that the Pusher buys, the Critic joins the team and criticizes us for not reading them, for not reading them carefully enough, for forgetting what we have read, or for not underlining properly.

The Critic works with the Pusher to get us to move, move, move! At any sign that we are getting too lazy, that we might possibly fall behind, that we might be less than the next person, the Critic will point out our failing to us and the Pusher will start to push. The Critic's cry, when it is teamed up with the Pusher, is: "You are just not making it. Everyone is out there ahead of you."

THE PERFECTIONIST

The Perfectionist is another common primary self that develops to help us succeed in the world. It wants us to look perfect, act perfect, and be perfect in all that we do. It will not tolerate a shoddy job and will drive us to distraction, redoing and redoing everything until it is just right. Nothing is less important than anything else. It is just as important to play perfectly during a friendly tennis volley as in the final match of a tournament. If something is worth doing, it is worth doing perfectly. And that is all there is to that. Perfect is perfect.

If our goal is perfection, then whose job is it to find the imperfections? You've guessed it, it is our friend, the Inner Critic! If the Perfectionist sets the standard of perfection, then the Critic will help us to achieve the goal, no matter how unrealistic or inappropriate it may be. There is no question about priorities; everything is equally important and everything must be just right. The Critic with its eagle eye and its superior intelligence will find every mistake, awkwardness, or problem and point it out to us with glee.

So, as you can see from these examples, our Inner Critic is not alone but will play ball with any of the primary selves that dominate our lives.

IF THESE ARE ALL SELVES, THEN WHO ARE WE?

Before we discover that we are made up of selves, we think that our primary selves are who we are. We think that the set of primary selves, the personality, that we have developed to protect us truly represents us. If I have a strong Perfectionist and a strong Pusher as two of my primary selves, I just assume that I am a perfectionistic and hardworking person, and that perhaps I'm even a bit driven.

Often we allow our lives to be run by our Rule Makers, Inner Critics, Pushers, Perfectionists, Pleasers, Responsible Parents, and other selves. When we do, no real choices are available to us. We must continue to live our lives by their rules. We call this collection of primary selves our *Operating Ego*. When this Operating Ego is in charge, we are not driving our own psychological cars. Instead, they are driven by whichever of our primary selves is the strongest at the moment. Our disowned selves, such as our Boundary Setters, our Fun Lovers, our

Daydreamers, our Self-Indulgent Princesses, our Warriors, our Incompetent Oafs, and our Irresponsible Children, are locked securely in the trunk.

INTRODUCING THE AWARE EGO

Once we become aware of our primary selves, we are able to begin to separate from them and to pick up the information and the feelings of the disowned selves on the opposite side. Or, to use the analogy of the car, we take over control of the car from the primary selves, rescue the disowned selves from the trunk, and drive our own psychological car with all of these selves as passengers. This is the position of an *Aware Ego*. It is only from an Aware Ego, when we have access to the opposites within us, that we have real choice about what we do in life. Then, and only then, are we in a position to truly care for ourselves.

The separation from your primary selves is the first step in developing an Aware Ego. This Aware Ego is not a self. It is a "you" that is not dominated by any self or set of selves. It is able to contain all the opposites that you are, to accept and to honor them appropriately. It moves you beyond duality. It is a process, not a goal. Your Aware Ego will not remain with you at all times because it disappears each time your primary selves take over. Your primary selves will automatically take to protect you when you are vulnerable. You can think of them as providing a much-needed safety net.

The Aware Ego gives you the ability to discover the complexity of your feelings and the richness of the many selves that inhabit your psyche. It also enables you to move in closer and closer to your own psychic fingerprint and to reclaim the unique human being that you were born to be. If you wish, you can read more about the Aware Ego in our previous writings.

In reading this book, you are doing a very important piece of work. You are separating from your Inner Critic, one of your primary selves, and developing an Aware Ego in relation to that particular self. As you do so, you no longer need to be the victim of your Inner Critic and you are able to operate from an Aware Ego in one very important aspect of your life—in evaluating yourself and your behavior.

> Stones' Warning: *Trying* to live life from an Aware Ego gives the Inner Critic the best food of all! Inner Critics simply love to accuse us of not having an Aware Ego. We all do the best that we can and each of us is in process. If you try too hard to live your life from an Aware Ego, it is a sure sign that your Pusher and/or Perfectionist have taken over again. This will allow your Inner Critic to grow even fatter as it tries to help you to reach this new, and unattainable, goal.

EXERCISES

The following are some questions for you to consider and exercises for you to do. We have included questions or exercises at the ends of chapters to help you experience within yourself the material covered in that specific chapter. They are also intended to help you become aware of and separate from your own Inner Critic. These exercises may be helpful to you, but they are certainly not essential requirements for getting the most out of this book. Take a look at them and see if you wish to consider them.

If you do decide to work on these exercises, you may wish to work with one or more other people. We have found that it can be very helpful, and often amusing, to hear how the Critic works in others. In addition, when one has a strong Critic, one's awareness and one's power to deal with the Critic is strengthened by the presence of other people who are doing the same work. If working on these exercises upsets you, please stop the work. You might even consider the possibility of professional help with this material if you find that your own Inner Critic has too much power in your life.

We have prepared three sets of exercises for this first chapter, and "Getting to Know Your Inner Critic" is the topic for the first set. We are going to try to help you learn how to tune in to radio station KRAZY so that you begin to hear what your own Critic is saying to you. As we have said, this is the first step in recognizing your Critic's voice and separating from it.

◆ GETTING TO KNOW YOUR INNER CRITIC

1. *Tuning in to Station KRAZY.* Over a one- to three-day period of time, pay attention to the critical things you say or feel about yourself. For example, you might be looking in the mirror, as you do every morning, and suddenly you become aware of how much time you spend looking disapprovingly at your face. Notice what you don't like about it. Pay attention to the things you say or feel about yourself that you take for granted. "I'm way too fat. I can't stand my hair. My nose is just too big!" When someone says that they can't stand something about themselves, it is not the person who is speaking. It is the Inner Critic that is speaking.

Later in the day, listen for your Critic when you are driving your car, waiting for an appointment, going to bed at night, waking up during the night, or waking up in the morning. Your Critic is there talking in your head all the time. Catch hold of it and listen to what it is saying. What does it think is wrong with you? What were the mistakes you made during the day? Where could you have done better? What have you overlooked? What should you have done differently?

The things that make you dissatisfied with yourself reflect the judgments of your Inner Critic. We have found that many people have an easier time catching hold of the Critic if they record its comments in a notebook. In this way, you begin to tune in to station KRAZY. Congratulations! It has been playing for years. You are now beginning to hear it clearly.

2. *Compare Your Station KRAZY with Others'.* Now compare notes with other people. What are some of the similarities and differences between the comments of your Critic and the Critics of other people? Talk to as many people as you possibly can because comparing your Inner Critic to others' begins to take the sting out of your own Inner Critic's comments which, up until

this time, have seemed accurate and specific to you alone. You will be surprised to find that others' Critics tell them the same things that yours tells you. You can easily see the exaggeration and inaccuracies of other people's Critics. This gives you additional power and objectivity. After all, you are not the only one who has these worries about yourself.

In getting together with others and sharing your Critics' comments—perhaps having a Critic Party—you have an opportunity to support one another in the process of separating from the Inner Critic. This can be much more fun than doing it alone. These sharings can even get hilarious, because Critics do have a way of getting pretty outrageous.

3. *What Does Your Critic Look Like?* Now that you have heard what your Inner Critic sounds like, we would like you to see what it looks like. The following exercise gives you a way to objectify your Inner Critic, to make it concrete, and to start to see it as a physical reality outside of yourself.

Take a piece of paper and draw a picture of your Inner Critic. If you prefer, make a clay model of it, or if you have no clay perhaps you would like to use Play-Doh or some other material that appeals to you. Use your imagination and remember that this is not a test of your artistic ability. Relax and have fun. There are no rules. Some Critics look like mothers or fathers or siblings. Some look like animals or dragons. Some look fierce, some do not. Some carry books in which to record your shortcomings. Each Inner Critic is unique. What does yours look like?

Now, if it is appropriate to you, give it a name. You may find that this is the name of someone near and dear to you whom your Critic resembles, like one of your parents or a teacher. Or it may have a name that is all its own. Giving the Critic a name is a further step in the process of making it more objective.

♦ WHERE DID YOUR CRITIC COME FROM?

In the following exercises you will have the opportunity to uncover the roots of your very own Critic. It did not originate in the heavens above, but it grew in the fertile soil provided by the judgments of the people around you. As you see the origin of your Inner Critic's favorite judgments, your Aware Ego grows in strength and objectivity.

1. In the first exercise, you already have recorded a number of statements made by your Inner Critic. Take each statement separately and ask yourself the following questions:

a. Does this statement sound like somebody I know? For example, if the statement is, "You are too bossy," this might be something your mother used to say to you. Pay particular attention to your parents, siblings, grandparents, uncles and aunts, teachers, and religious leaders.

b. When do I first remember being concerned about this issue? This may be difficult, but sometimes a particular incident or period in life was so painful that the Critic jumped in quite suddenly to "help."

2. Write down your mother's favorite judgmental comments about you. If she did not say these out loud, what was it about you that you knew displeased her?

3. Think of the ways in which your mother judged other people. Write down some of her favorite judgments about others.

4. Write down some judgmental comments that your father made about you when he criticized you. If he did not say these out loud, what was it about you that you knew displeased him?

5. Think of the ways in which your father judged other people. Write down his favorite judgments of others.

6. What were the worst characteristics that a person could have, according to your grade school classmates?

7. What were the worst characteristics that a person could have, according to your high school classmates?

8. What were the worst characteristics that a person could have, according to your college classmates?

9. What are the worst characteristics that a person could have, according to your current friends?

Now you can see the origin of some of the most popular scripts used on your special station KRAZY. You are beginning to gain some separation from your Inner Critic.

♦ STRENGTHENING THE AWARE EGO: DISCOVERING THE PRIMARY AND DISOWNED SELVES

The following exercises will help you to discover your own primary and disowned self systems. This is fascinating work and of the utmost importance in developing an Aware Ego that can be truly objective.

1. In order to discover your primary selves, you begin by looking for your disowned selves. There is a simple, straightforward way for you to discover these selves because the people whom we judge and dislike are carrying our disowned selves.

Think of somebody in your life whom you really do not like, somebody who pushes your emotional buttons. This should be someone who makes you feel self-righteous and superior. Get a clear picture of this person. What is it about this person that you really judge? When you figure this out, you have discovered a disowned self.

For instance, you might dislike your mother-in-law. As you think about what it is that you particularly dislike, you realize that she is very needy and she wants others to take care of her. You would never, ever want to be like that! This, then, is your disowned self. You have disowned your needy child who wants others to take care of her.

Now, on to the discovery of your primary self. Your primary self is the opposite of your disowned self. To continue with our example, you would think of how you are opposite in character to your mother-in-law. You, in contrast to her, are self-sufficient and would never think of asking anyone for attention or help. You are independent, you take care of yourself, and you are proud of it. Thus, one of your most important primary selves is an Independent Self.

This next step is optional. Now that you have discovered your primary self, your Independent Self who really does not need anyone else, you might want to imagine at what point in your life it was born and how it served to protect you, and particularly the Vulnerable Child in you. Perhaps your family was chaotic and there was really nobody that you could depend upon. This independent, self-sufficient self would have figured out how you could make it through life on your own. It would have protected you. Or perhaps your mother was needy, nobody respected her, and she was a victim to your father and to the world in general. It was apparent that neediness was not safe, so a primary self that was independent and self-sufficient developed to protect your Vulnerable Child and keep you strong.

2. The second way that you can discover a disowned self is by looking at someone you overvalue. The people whom you overvalue, the ones who make you feel inferior, carry your disowned selves.

Think of someone you overvalue. This is not someone you just admire, but someone who makes you feel bad about yourself in comparison. Again you will have discovered a disowned self.

Perhaps you admire your best friend's ability to be rational and in control. You, in contrast, always seem to get emotional and confused when something is important to you. You wish that you could be calm, cool, and collected like she is. In fact, when you are with her, or even think about her, you seem to get more emotional and confused than usual. She is showing you a disowned self. You have disowned your own rational, controlled part.

Now, look for your primary self. How is it that you are opposites? You are far more emotional. Your primary self is emotional and not controlled.

Again, if you wish, move on to the next step. Why do you think you developed such a primary self? Perhaps that is the way your entire family was. Emotions were admired and encouraged, and being in control was judged as constricted and uptight. Or perhaps one of your parents was so cold and controlled that you did not want to be like that and your development moved in the opposite direction.

3. Now that you have begun to separate from your primary selves, you will make an interesting discovery about your Inner Critic. One of your Inner Critic's major tasks in life is to support these primary selves and to criticize anything that has to do with your disowned selves. Therefore, the value system of your primary selves has been determining the specific content of your Critic's judgments. Thus, as you separate from your primary selves and develop an Aware Ego, fewer judgments are necessary to support your primary-self system and you will find that your Critic begins to lose some of its power.

Chapter Two

_____

How We Talk to the Inner Critic

Another thing that we discovered in talking to the selves in each other was the sense of their absolute reality. The Inner Child, the Inner Critic, the Responsible Parent—each of these was no longer just a part or subpersonality in our minds. They gradually emerged on the canvas of our psyches as real, live people, and the more that we explored, the more amazed we became. What started out as a coexploration between us became, ultimately, the method that we have called Voice Dialogue.

You have learned about the fact that we are made up of different selves. You are beginning to get some feel for how these selves develop and how important it is to learn about their ways of operating in your life. Early in our own relationship with each other we needed to find a way to explore ourselves and to help each other in this exploration. It was out of this need to more deeply understand ourselves and to deepen our own relationship that we began to talk to the different selves in each other. We took turns "facilitating" each other. (Facilitating means talking to the other person's selves.) In those early days, we spent hundreds of hours discovering the amazingly widespread and rich family of selves that lived inside of each of us.

When it was Sidra's turn to be subject, Hal would first spend some time talking with her to see what kinds of issues she wanted to deal with. Once there was a sense of what self or selves needed to be dealt with, he would ask her to change her physical position, to actually move to the place where that self or voice was sitting. Hal then would begin a dialogue with this particular voice. Having a dialogue with a voice means that Hal would begin to talk to a particular voice in Sidra and that voice would talk back to Hal. From this in-depth conversation the voice received the opportunity to express its feelings and ideas in great detail. These dialogues might last only five or ten minutes, or they might go on for one or two hours.

When it was Hal's turn to be subject, the procedure would be reversed. Sidra would be the facilitator and she would ask Hal to move over to the place where a specific self (like the Pusher) would sit. She would then carry on a conversation with that particular voice. After this dialogue ended, Hal would move back to his original chair. From this position, it would be possible to view and experience the different selves that had emerged in the facilitation process.

In the course of these dialogues, no attempt is made to change the view or feelings of the different parts or selves. If two selves have different viewpoints, no attempt is made to have them talk to each other or become friends with one another. In this way, both the subject and the facilitator have an opportunity to learn how to live with the many paradoxes of life.

After each of these sessions was over, we found that we were able to become much more separated from and objective about the different selves in us. We learned to honor all of them. The idea was not to try to get rid of parts that we did not like, something we had both tried to do for years. The idea was to embrace all of them and learn to use all of them with a new kind of awareness. That is how we developed the idea of the Aware Ego. The Aware Ego is the part of us that is always changing as it becomes more aware of and experiences the different selves and then gradually learns how to use them in life with real choice.

We learned too that the more we tried to make a part go away, the stronger it became. We discovered that there were many people who recognized the Inner Critic, for example, and who were always trying to make it go away because they hated it so much. The more they would try to rid themselves of the Critic, the stronger it would grow inside. The trick, we learned, was to let the parts speak, to understand who they were and how they developed, and to learn how to use them properly in life.

Another thing that we discovered in working with each other was how real these selves were. As we have said, they behave as though they are real people, each with its own hopes, feelings, and ambitions. Most of them have a real sense of how we should live our lives. What was different about our experience with each other from our prior experience was this sense of their absolute reality. The Inner Child, the Inner Critic, the Responsible Parent—each of these was no longer just a part or subpersonality. They were real, live people to us, and the more we explored, the more amazed we became. What started out as coexploration between us became ultimately the method that we have called Voice Dialogue. We have described this method in considerable detail in our book *Embracing Our Selves,* and we refer the interested reader to this book for a full discussion of the method and the theory.

The reason that we bring this to your attention now is that in this book on the Inner Critic we will be using Voice Dialogue to show you conversations that we have had with the Inner Critic. You will have a chance to read about how the Critic feels and sounds and the kinds of things that it is saying constantly inside the minds of people. The more that you hear and read about the voice of the Inner Critic, the easier it will be to hear your own Critic and to begin the ever-important process of separating from it.

Keep in mind, then, the basic procedure of Voice Dialogue from which these conversations come. The "subject" is the one whose inner selves are speaking. The "facilitator" is guiding the dialogue. The facilitator asks the subject to physically move to the place where the Inner Critic (or other self) is sitting. The facilitator then begins to talk to the Critic, and a dialogue ensues between Critic and facilitator. We will be citing portions of these dialogues throughout the rest of this book.

VOICE DIALOGUE AS A WAY TO WORK WITH THE INNER CRITIC

As you can see, Voice Dialogue is an excellent way of getting to know your Inner Critic directly by talking to it. In addition to this, we believe that Voice Dialogue is an extremely effective method for exploring and eventually coming to grips with the Inner Critic. As with any approach to personal growth, Voice Dialogue is not necessarily appropriate for everyone and must be seen in the context of all the psychospiritual work that you do. Voice Dialogue is a way of working that can be integrated into any growth-enhancing or therapeutic system. It is not designed to replace anything but rather to add a richness to whatever it is that you are now doing.

T W O

How the Inner Critic Operates

Chapter Three

The Critic as the Speaker
of Absolute Truth

So often when the Critic speaks to us it is as though a sin has been
committed, a crime has been perpetrated, or a dark and evil deed
has been done. The Critic does not simply give opinions or express
feelings about things. Its statements become a judgment from
heaven above.

When the Inner Critic speaks to us, it does so in a particular
way. It makes pronouncements. It does not simply give opinions or express feelings about things. It makes absolute pronouncements. It sounds as though a voice from the heavens is
handing down absolute truths to us—something like the Ten
Commandments. This ability to make itself sound like absolute
truth is one of the reasons that the Critic is so difficult to deal
with. The major problem in dealing with the Critic is, of course,
the fact that most of us do not have the foggiest notion that it is
speaking to us. Even when we are aware of its voice, we usually have no separation from it because it sounds like it has the
truth of heaven behind it.

For example, let us go back to the peanut butter party that we
spoke about in chapter 1. The Critic says to our midnight
snacker, "You are a slob. You do not have an ounce of control
and you never will." If the snacker happens to be in the field of
health and healing, the Critic might add, "And you are supposed
to be helping people? I cannot believe you!" The fundamental
doctrine that is being advanced by the Critic is as follows:

1. You have no business eating at night.
2. You should have perfect control at all times.
3. Normal people would not do this.
4. A health care professional, in particular, should have more control.
5. Problems of any kind are bad.

A sin has been committed. A crime has been perpetrated. A dark and evil deed has been done. The effect of this kind of statement is profound. You feel like a slob. You become a slob. You feel out of control. It does not matter that you have control in a hundred other areas. It does not matter that you have clear boundaries at work or in many of your relationships. It does not matter that you did not eat the peanut butter and jelly sandwich the night before. You become the slob and the out-of-control person that your Critic says you are. Its comments become a kind of judgment from heaven above.

For women, this judgment often has to do with their sexual attractiveness. Marie awakens in the morning, looks in the mirror, sees her body, and in particular her breasts, and she feels a sense of profound negativity about them. She believes that they are too small. Her Inner Critic, for that of course is who the culprit is, compares her breasts constantly to other women, and in every case her breasts are found inferior. The conclusion that her Critic reaches is that she will never be truly attractive to a man.

Using the Voice Dialogue method, we have a conversation with her Inner Critic because we want to help Marie to hear this voice and to begin separating from it. We ask Marie to move over to the place where the Inner Critic is sitting, and, as we described in the previous chapter, we begin to talk to the Critic directly.

FACILITATOR: It seems that you have some very negative feelings about Marie's body.

INNER CRITIC: Well, quite frankly, I think she has a terrible body.

FACILITATOR: Could you tell me what you don't like?

INNER CRITIC: Well, quite frankly, I don't like anything about her body. She's much too thin. HER FRAME IS WRONG! She just has a wrong frame. Nothing fits together properly.

FACILITATOR: She mentioned being very sensitive about her breasts. I assume that it is you who criticizes them.

INNER CRITIC: Well, like I told you, she has a wrong frame. The rest follows. Nothing works. Her breasts are terrible because they're too small! They sag! Just look at her. Anyone can see that. Just look at her. It's obvious to anyone who looks at her. Can't you tell?

FACILITATOR: Not really. She looks fine to me, but then I'm not her Critic. That's your job.

CRITIC: WELL, YOU SHOULD SEE HER NAKED! (A favorite expression of the Critic.) THEN YOU WOULD UNDERSTAND! (Pronouncement complete.)

It is not just the words that matter when the Inner Critic speaks. It is the quality of energy behind these words. This is why we have capitalized a few of these comments. So powerful are these statements and so deeply into the psyche do they go that Marie experiences herself as having a wrong frame whenever she looks in the mirror. When she goes shopping she will have a terrible time because she has a frame that is all wrong and there is nothing she can try on that will work for her. Her Critic has spoken!

So powerful are these kinds of judgments that many people we know have literally stopped looking in mirrors because what they saw was simply too unattractive for them to tolerate. It is as though they are wearing Inner Critic glasses and everything about themselves is seen through these lenses. A piece of the shattered glass of our hobgoblin's mirror (described in chapter 1) has penetrated the eyes of our poor victim, and everything about her looks terrible. Often when we try to help people separate from the Critic, someone will say to us, "But it's true, what the

Critic says is true, my breasts really *are* too small!" The absolute truth is known. The Critic has spoken. So for the rest of her life, Marie walks around with a sense of total inadequacy about her body.

What is particularly amazing is that these pronouncements have little to do with objective reality. A hundred people could tell Marie that her body is lovely and really mean it. The Critic will have none of this, and it is this critical perspective that will prevail so long as Marie has not separated from these internal judgments.

The judgments of the Critic about our moral imperfections can be even more devastating. When the Inner Critic tells us that we should be ashamed of ourselves—our actions, thoughts, or impulses—and its comments are backed up with that sound of absolute authority, we cringe. We just know that we cannot defend ourselves and we are deeply shamed.

When we consider issues of low self-esteem and shame, we generally try to understand where they came from. This understanding of the past is certainly essential work for our personal growth. We can, however, also deal with the present. We can become aware of the fact that the Inner Critic is operating inside of us right now! We can begin to see how much of our low self-esteem and sense of shame and depression is a function of this Critic who has learned from so many different sources how to do its job.

What a boon to our personal growth it would be to recognize this critical voice as a voice, nothing more and nothing less, and to be able to deal with it in an objective way! *The ability to separate from the Inner Critic and no longer be dominated by its negative injunctions will result in a major shift in one's sense of self-esteem and self-worth*. Can there be a better motivation for doing this work?

When you hear and read about the voice of the Inner Critic a hundred times, a thousand times, then you begin to get some perspective on this matter. The job of the Inner Critic is to criticize. The more we are victims of its absolute judgments, the more power it gets. The size of the breast is really not an objective issue. If you separate from the Critic and decide your breasts are fine, then it will point out that something is wrong with the way you raise your children. It will tell you that you are too selfish or too giving. It will tell you that you are a bad father or husband or wife or mother. It will let you know that you are not really a good friend. The Critic does not care about your breasts. It cares about criticizing. Criticism is its lifeblood. In Voice Dialogue conversations it will often say to the facilitator, "But what could I possibly do if I did not criticize him?"

If we were going to express this as a kind of universal principle, it would go something like this. *The sense of authority, purpose, and meaning that we lack in our own lives is often carried by the Inner Critic.* The lack of awareness that we have of our different selves, and in particular the Inner Critic, provides a playground and feeding lot on which the Inner Critic can develop and grow into the heavenly emissary it has become within most of us.

As you read this, you are already learning to separate from the Inner Critic and learning to handle it so that you are no longer under its domination. In the course of your personal development, as you take back the authority and purpose of your life that is rightfully yours, you develop a capacity for awareness that is decisively greater than the original power of the Critic. With this new power and authority available to you, you have the possibility of redeeming the Inner Critic so that it can begin to function in a very different way in your life, a way that supports who and what you are. The realization that your Inner Critic is not a heavenly emissary speaking absolute truths is a great step forward in taking back this power.

Chapter Four

The Critic's View of the Physical Body

We are bombarded in our culture by specialness. Beng ordinary is simply not acceptable. The demands of physical perfection are like a runaway train that we could call the Special Express. It is no wonder that the Critic has developed so much power when it comes to judging our physical bodies.

We have had conversations with literally thousands of Inner Critics during the past fifteen years. We have heard them criticize just about everything there is to criticize in a human being. We doubt that there is much that could surprise us at this point. The critique of the physical body is so all-pervasive, so powerful, and exerts such a negative and destructive influence on people's lives that we want to devote a chapter specifically to this area of the Critic's function.

GENERAL CONSIDERATIONS

People are always saying that they don't like this or that about their bodies. They will say such things as, "I don't like the shape of my face. My hips are too big. My neck is too short. My hair just lies there like a wet dishrag. My toes are crooked. I cannot stand the way my ears stick out." It never occurs to most people that these negative feelings about their bodies do not belong to them as aware human beings. Similarly, it never occurs to them that these are comments made by the Inner Critic. Most of us take this abuse for granted and when we use the word *I* as we describe our perceptions of our physical bodies, we actually mean the perceptions of our Inner Critics.

FALLING IN LOVE

In the kind of situation described above, when there is no Aware Ego and when someone is fully identified with the Inner Critic, no amount of reassurance will help. If you tell such a person that her hair is really lovely, the Critic will counter that with a comment such as, "She's just trying to make you feel good" or, "She says that to everyone." Or if you tell such a woman that her blouse looks great on her, she will feel quite embarrassed because her Critic will be saying in her head, "He should know what you really look like." As we have pointed out before, the Inner Critic's comments are like a mantra, repeating over and over in your head: "The trouble with you is. The trouble with you is . . . ! The trouble with you is . . . !" There is no way to counter this from the outside, and it generally is present except for one period of time in people's lives, and that is when they fall in love.

During the falling-in-love period, with the accompanying joy of romantic love, these Inner Critics generally fall asleep for a period of time. The other person loves us unconditionally and we love him or her unconditionally. Our Inner Children flower and feel safe and the garden grows because there is no one around to stomp on it. Having someone love you unconditionally and having this person's full attention focused upon you is a soporific for the Inner Critic. Whereas you may always have been very critical of your eyes (the Critic told you they were too close together and the wrong color), your partner adores them, and suddenly your eyes are beautiful. The world truly sparkles because all the negative evaluations are gone.

As this phase of the relationship comes to an end, however, the Inner Critic returns. Your partner who has loved your eyes unreservedly and who has given you full-time attention now gets busy at work again. He or she still loves you, but that total commitment is not there in the same way. He is back into himself and the intense romantic involvement is waning. Maybe she even has reactions that she is not sharing and these, of course, become judgments. You may even find yourself responding at some level to these unconscious feelings.

As the romantic phase ends and as the constant positive feedback ends, the Critic returns and lets you know again that your eyes are spaced too closely together. Your partner may try to reassure you that this is not true, but somehow this does not sound the same as before and your partner no longer has the power to hold back the renewed onslaught of the Critic.

SOME SOURCES OF THE CRITIC'S POWER

This critique of the physical body causes people enormous pain. As we mentioned in the last chapter, we have seen many instances of people who simply refuse to look into mirrors because they cannot bear what they see there. This may come as a surprise to you, but the Inner Critic has a number of very special places where it lives and rests. You will learn more about these later in this chapter. For the moment we will simply share with you the fact that one of its special resting places is bathroom mirrors. It loves to live inside these mirrors and look back at you when you look into it. The next time you look in the mirror, look carefully and deeply behind the glass and you will see him or her peering out at you.

For many people clothes shopping is a nightmare because nothing possibly could look good on them. A number of years ago Hal met with a young actress who was quite beautiful. In talking with her Inner Critic, however, one would have thought that a monster was sitting across from him. He (her Critic was a he) ripped her apart. There was nothing right with her body. Shopping was a total nightmare for her. She was devastated and lived as painful victim to this judgmental self inside her. Being an actress could not change a lifetime of criticism and judgment from her parents. She had long since broken with them, but on the inner level they were stronger than ever. No amount of objective validation could make any difference. A very strong

Inner Critic turned the world into a system of judgments, all directed toward her, spoken or unspoken.

We have described how these Critics develop in us. They come from parents, siblings, school, religious leaders, books, everyone in our environment. One time Hal was facilitating the Inner Critic of a woman and she started laughing and could hardly stop. What Diane had remembered was an incident with her mother just before her mother died. Diane recalled that her mother was exceptionally critical. At the time of this incident her mother was eighty-five years of age and was in a hospital suffering from a terminal illness. She had great difficulty breathing, and it was obvious that the end was near. Diane walked into the hospital room on this particular morning, and the mother, who had been semicomatose for several days, saw her enter the room. She suddenly sat up in bed and said to her daughter: "Is that the only purse you have?" She then collapsed back into her coma and died a few hours later. This kind of judgment obviously leads to very strong Inner Critics.

We have noticed a clear pattern: *The stronger the Inner Critic, the stronger the judgmental voices that have been around the person in the growing-up process. The stronger the judgmental voices around us in the growing-up process, the stronger will be the Inner Critic.*

A CONVERSATION WITH THE CRITIC
ABOUT ANNIE'S BODY

We are going to give you now a longer Voice Dialogue conversation, though still an excerpt, with an Inner Critic that is sharing its feelings about Annie. This particular Critic was quite powerful, so we decided to focus first on the body itself and then move on into other areas.

FACILITATOR (to Critic): Since you seem to have so much to criticize Annie about, why don't we do it in some kind of wholistic fashion and start first with the physical body? I know from what Annie has said so far that you don't like a lot of things about her body.

CRITIC: What's to like? Look at her. Just look at her!

FACILITATOR: Well, I am looking. Quite honestly, she looks pretty good to me.

CRITIC: You're just trying to make her feel good. There is so much wrong I don't know where to start.

FACILITATOR: Let's do it scientifically. We'll start with her hair and you can rate each part on a hundred-point scale where zero is the worst and one hundred is the best. Let's start with her hair. How would you rate that?

CRITIC: I'd give it a ten or twenty.

FACILITATOR: What is wrong with it? Why so low?

CRITIC: Well, first of all, it has no luster. It's dry. It's too short. I don't like the color. She never does anything with it. She might be okay if she lived in Africa in some village.

FACILITATOR: What about her face?

CRITIC: It's too plain. There is no character to it. Her nose is too large and it's too compacted. I don't like her complexion either. She always looks like she's on the verge of hepatitis.

FACILITATOR: You really are rough on her. What is your rating?

CRITIC: I'll give it a twenty.

FACILITATOR: You're coming in pretty low so far, aren't you?

CRITIC: You asked me how I feel about her. I'm only speaking the truth.

FACILITATOR: How do you feel about her shoulders?

CRITIC: Actually, they're not so bad. I'd give them a fifty.

FACILITATOR: If they're not so bad, why does she only get a fifty?

CRITIC: She gets nothing over a fifty because she doesn't deserve anything over a fifty.

FACILITATOR: What about the shape of her body in general?

CRITIC: You have got to be kidding! Do you have a week to spend on this? Her body is a horror story. Look at her hips. They're huge. And her thighs. Aside from being too large she has cellulite. I've told her a hundred times to have the cellulite taken off. (It is amazing how many Inner Critics are cellulite experts.) She won't listen to me. So I keep at her.

FACILITATOR: Could anything she ever did satisfy you? Truthfully now, could she ever get you to stop criticizing her?

CRITIC: Not really. She's just weak. She lets me criticize her and never even thinks of stopping me. She deserves everything that she gets.

FACILITATOR: Where did you learn how to be such a powerful Critic? It seems as though you've had some very good schooling.

CRITIC: Oh, I had the best schooling of all. Her mother had a Ph.D. in judgment. Her father only had a B.A. in judgment. Then her older sister got her Ph.D. in judgment, and I learned from all of them. She could never do anything right. Anything she wore was wrong and her body was simply something that needed to be fixed. I had the best of training. To tell you the truth, I started criticizing her so that she would be prepared for their attacks. I figured that if I got to her first, it might not hurt as much when they went after her.

It is amazing how often one hears the Inner Critic attack someone for being too weak to stop it. That is one of the paradoxes of the Inner Critic. It pounds us and pounds us, and in this process it hates us for being so weak. It actually criticizes us for having an Inner Critic that is out of control.

The Voice Dialogue excerpt that we have given to you is only an excerpt. The kinds of things that the Critic can find wrong with our physical bodies are infinite in variety. It can often go on for hours.

When facilitating, we sometimes ask what appear to be silly and outlandish questions. Then the Aware Ego can hear how far-out, how absolutely extreme, the Critic is in its judgments toward us.

For example, we might ask the Critic such things as, "How do you feel about John's big toe or Mary's right kneecap or Al's earlobe or Yvonne's elbow or the hair on Harry's chest?" Invariably the Critic will have something negative and quite reasonable to say about whatever it is we are asking about. This amazing power of the Critic to attack us in this way causes great suffering and anguish in people. Low self-esteem does not even begin to describe the shape that Annie is in because of these constant Critic attacks and evaluations. What chance does she have to make a successful relationship with these kinds of self-evaluations constantly going on in her? Such Critics create victims, and such victims have a very difficult time feeling equal to other people.

People's identification with the Critic is often so complete that they will say to us, "But what he says is true. My hair *is* terrible. I *am* too short. My thighs *are* too big." To remain identified with this Critic is to live in prison. To separate from it—to recognize that these critiques are coming from a voice, from a person who lives inside of you—is to leave this dungeon of despair. The conversation we have given you is just a plain, ordinary, everyday dialogue. There is nothing special or unique about it. It is going on in the heads of people much of the time. We must realize that radio station KRAZY is playing in our heads. Once we know this we can change the station or turn off the radio.

THE "TALKING" BATHROOM SCALE AND MIRROR

No discussion of the Critic's view of the physical body would be complete without consideration of the talking bathroom scale and the talking mirror that we alluded to earlier in this chapter. Most people are not aware of the talking scale in their homes. Every time you step onto it or look into it, a voice speaks out. (There are actually scales that talk to you, telling you your weight and comparing it to what it was yesterday. What a joy for your Inner Critic! What we are talking about here, however, is the commentary of your Critic that only you can hear.) Similarly, every time you look into the mirror, you hear comments, marvelous comments, such as,

Oh my God! I can't believe your weight (or face)!

Look at the lines on your face!

Please put on your make-up!

I told you to skip dessert last night!

It was pig-out time again! (Variation on this one:) You're bloated!

Your hair is dead!

If you were going to the gym regularly this wouldn't happen!

When are you ever going to lose weight!

What more can we say? We know that there are positive features of scales and mirrors and reasons why we need them. Certainly, however, for the Inner Critic the bathroom scale and the bathroom mirror are the greatest inventions since the wheel. It is a morning ritual that is more powerful than coffee and one that ensures the Critic a major say in how our morning begins each day. Or should we say, how our mourning begins each day?

SPECIAL NOURISHMENT FOR THE CRITIC

It is easy to see how the Critic is nourished by judgmental parents and siblings and other persons in our environment. Add to this Critic soup pot the magazines: *Playboy, Playgirl, Vogue, Harpers Bazaar, GQ, Body Building,* and a multitude of other magazines that sing the praises of how to be one of the "beautiful people." Add a few cups of weight reduction clinics and aerobics classes. Add fourteen gallons of television and movie images constantly showing us the "most attractive" men, women, body, legs, hair. Even *plain* in television means glamorous.

To this we must add five bushels of advertising that constantly put in front of us women models who weigh ninety-six pounds and men who are built like Arnold Schwarzenegger or dressed to the hilt, and unbelievably suave and debonair, in gorgeous Italian suits. Add two quarts of sexy, passionate love scenes that show unbelievable lovemaking done by the greatest pros in the business. Add our final ingredient: several gallons of an elixir called "being special." This is a very nourishing soup that our Critics are fed every day of our lives. It is no wonder that the Critic has so much clout when it comes to judging our physical bodies.

There is one ingredient that is not allowed in this Critic soup. It is a criminal act to introduce the ingredient of normal or ordinary. Our culture has become a runaway train that we would have to call the Special Express. So much of the input that we receive has to do with being special. Watching a jeans commercial on television raises the rear end of people to a status approaching divinity.

Lovemaking is never ordinary or boring on television or films. Certainly filmmakers must have experienced or heard about just an ordinary, average kiss or lovemaking session. Does anyone ever kiss without musical accompaniment? Is it any wonder that the Critic goes berserk in the face of all of this and demands some mythical, special, nonordinary way of being in the world? For a woman to strive toward the ideal form of a fourteen-year-old and for a man to strive toward the ideal form of a weight lifter or hard-as-steel cop is unrealistic, to say the least. All of this contributes toward the massive power that the Inner Critic has achieved in so many people. It would be funny if it did not cause so many people such grief.

◆ HOW DOES YOUR CRITIC VIEW YOUR BODY?

1. Gather together a large number of different magazines and look at the advertisements that use male and female models.

What is your impression of them and how do they affect you? Tune in to your Inner Critic's comments as you look at them.

2. What do you remember in growing up about being special and ordinary? Were you pushed in a certain direction? Who pushed you and why?

3. How does your Critic feel about the possibility of your being just ordinary? What does it say about this?

4. What does your Inner Critic like to criticize about your physical body? Does it do this by comparing you to other people?

5. Do you have a talking scale? What does it say in the morning?

6. Do you have a talking bathroom mirror? What does it say in the morning to you?

Chapter Five

The Wholistic Critic
A Self-Improvement Expert

In all of the learning that we do in relation to personal growth, we have a partner. The Critic would call itself an ally. It is with us when we read a book or attend a lecture. It is with us at every seminar that we take, and it listens to every conversation we have. It soaks up information like a dry sponge. It is operating right now as you read this book, and it will use this information in some way to criticize you.

One of the first things to appreciate about the Inner Critic is that it is by nature wholistic. It criticizes everything about us with equal enthusiasm. It criticizes our bodies, our emotions, our minds, and our spirituality. In the old days, before we all became involved in personal growth, its sphere of influence and its available power were somewhat limited. What is important to realize about the Inner Critic as it operates in most of us today is that it has grown up in the New Age of psychology and it has absorbed an amazing amount of information about the way we should and should not be.

As we have seen, the Critic works closely with the Rule Maker, the Pusher, and the Perfectionist, three very important selves in us. The Rule Maker is the person who figures out the way we should be in the world in order to make things safe for us. The Perfectionist sees that we do it properly. The Pusher jams us to see that things are done right away and that we keep doing more and more things. The Critic then plays off these

three selves and criticizes us when it feels that we are not playing the game correctly, which is most of the time.

OUR PARTNER IN LEARNING

In all of the learning that we do in relation to personal growth,
we have a partner. It is with us when we read a book or attend
a lecture. It is with us in every seminar that we take and every
conversation that we have. It soaks up information like a dry
sponge. It is operating right now as you read this book, and it
will use this information in some way to criticize you. It may tell
you that you are not aware enough or that you are not bright
enough to understand this material. It may even criticize you for
having an Inner Critic. Let us look at an example of a Voice
Dialogue conversation to see how the Critic operates in relationship to personal growth.

Steve is a lovely young man who has become deeply involved
in personal growth work. He has read a good deal and attended
many lectures and workshops. What he has not realized, as we
have mentioned above, is the fact that the Inner Critic has been
with him attending all of the seminars and reading all of the
books. Let us see now what his Critic has to say about his work.
Keep in mind that all of these examples are taken from longer
Voice Dialogue conversations.

FACILITATOR: It sounds as though you enjoy a lot of the self-
help work that Steve does as much as he enjoys it.

CRITIC: I do. It gives me a great deal of information to think
about that I don't ordinarily have.

FACILITATOR: What, for example?

CRITIC: Well, I'm very interested in his eating since he got into
all of this nutritional work. His diet is terrible. I knew nothing about food before we started reading the new health
books. The class that he attended was fantastic. You know
how important nutrition is. I have to keep telling him to clean
up his act around food. I'm there whenever he eats, trying to

get him to do what's right. I've started to tell him how bad meat is. I tell him that he's eating dead animals. The trouble is that he likes meat.

FACILITATOR: And you apparently have a clear sense of what is right and what is wrong?

CRITIC: Well, that's why we read these books. All of these experts seem to know what is right, and I use that information. It's confusing sometimes because different experts say different things.

FACILITATOR: What else do you criticize?

CRITIC: He should be running every day, at least five miles a day. And he should be going to the gym.

FACILITATOR: Would that satisfy you?

CRITIC: I don't know. There's always more. He has to stretch. I don't want him to turn rigid. He needs more discipline about these things. I'd also like to see him start running meditatively. He read an article by someone about that and I thought that would be a good idea.

FACILITATOR: Is there anything else that is particularly important to you about Steve?

CRITIC: There's so much. I want him to write his dreams down every morning and also to start to meditate every morning. And he drinks coffee. I tell him to stop drinking coffee. It's a drug.

Steve's Critic and Pusher have combined to focus on his exercise and health routine with a little journal work thrown in. The list of *shoulds* can become amazingly long. Every *should* gives the Critic its opening. People are driven crazy by these kinds of requirements and attacks. Life itself ceases to be fun as the New Age Pusher and Critic lead people into this merry-go-round of New Age consciousness. It is not that the ideas themselves are bad. It is that they have an energy behind them that is very powerful and all-knowing and there is often too little discrimination and choice being made about what truly is appropriate for a person.

To understand the attacks of the Critic, we must keep in mind the underlying vulnerability and anxiety of this self. If we read a book and it tells us that something is bad for us, and if we do not have a strong enough Aware Ego to read this kind of statement and evaluate it properly, then it stirs up a miniature anxiety attack in us. The things that we learn from books, lectures, and workshops become the shoulds and shouldn'ts from which the Inner Critic gets its power. The bottom line for the Critic is that it wants us to be safe, successful, and economically protected. It wants to be sure that we are not abandoned, that we do not look foolish or do anything to embarrass ourselves in such a way that will cause abandonment. It is also terrified about our becoming ill because this means danger and the possibility of economic deprivation. For the Inner Critic, if we can but follow the shoulds and shouldn'ts of the Rule Maker and the Perfectionist, then everything will be okay and we will be safe.

The Critic remembers all too well the pain of our childhood, the innumerable times when we were shamed and criticized and made fun of. It remembers the anxiety of our parents about money. It still feels, through the feelings of the Inner Child, the terror of abandonment when we were left alone or when a divorce or separation caused a parent to leave. It desperately wants us to avoid that primal pain, and the only way it can handle it is to make us perfect. To make us perfect, it must criticize us because it has no other way to help us. Inner Critics do not come to us and say, "I'm feeling vulnerable and anxious and upset." We have to learn how to do that for them, and we have to realize that these are always the underlying issues, no matter how vicious the attack on us. It is only by understanding this underlying dynamic of the Critic that we can make sense about the nature of its attacks.

A CRITIC WITH A SPIRITUAL FOCUS

Jane is also involved in much personal growth work, but her focus is more on being spiritual and loving. She was always a very caring and loving child, and her entry into the spiritual movement enhanced this. Thus she has identified with a set of rules that says she must be caring and loving at all times and that this is the goal of spiritual development. The stage is set for her Inner Critic. Listen to the following Voice Dialogue conversation:

FACILITATOR: So far you have had a good deal to say about Jane in many different areas—all critical, I might add.

CRITIC: Well, that's my job. Without me she would be nowhere. She wouldn't amount to anything.

FACILITATOR: How do you feel about her spiritual development? You haven't said anything about that so far.

CRITIC: Well, the best I can say for her is that she tries. She has a long, long way to go, I can tell you that. I hardly know where to start. First of all, she doesn't meditate enough, and she gets distracted too easily. That bothers me. She sits there, and much of the time she is thinking about a hundred other things than what she is supposed to be doing. The worst thing, though, is that she gets upset too easily. She gets angry at her children and yells at them. Then she feels guilty and apologizes. She should have more control. If she were really spiritual she wouldn't have to get upset so much. It happens with her husband too. She's always getting angry with him about something or other. I really let her have it then.

FACILITATOR: It sounds like you would like Jane to be perfect. Never getting angry is a tall order.

CRITIC: It's just a matter of control. She grew up with a mother who was always flying into rages. We made up our mind early on that she would never be like that. She was the victim of that rage. There is no reason to perpetrate it on her children or anyone else. Besides that, it just isn't part of a spiritual tradition to be getting angry and emotional all the time.

Jane's Critic/Rule Maker combination was born out of re-action to an emotionally explosive mother. They became very central to her life, and they wanted her way of being in the world to be the opposite of her mother's explosive behavior. So the Critic has available a well-laid-out game plan. She makes sure that she reminds Jane whenever there is a loss of control. Of course, the emotional explosiveness grows inside of Jane and ultimately can damage her greatly. This is exactly the basis of much physical illness in people. The Critic does not mean to hurt her. It is just doing the job that it was trained to do.

THE INNER CRITIC AND THE RULE MAKER

It is clear from this conversation that in order to understand the Inner Critic, we must understand the system of rules under which a person operates in the world. The rules under which Jane operates are as follows.

1. One must be loving at all times.
2. Anger is bad.
3. In particular, anger at one's children is terrible.
4. In meditation one should be free of all extraneous thought.
5. One's marriage should be basically loving at all times.

Think of the consequences of these rules. It is like saying to someone, "Stand in the corner and do not think of an elephant!" Try as you may, you *will* think of an elephant, and the harder you try, the harder it will be to get the elephant out of your head. Try to be loving all the time, and you will be engorged with negativity. Try always to keep your mind clear while med-itating, and you will be invaded by thoughts and fantasies. Try always to be loving to your children, and you will be invaded periodically by negative feelings that will assault you. The more shoulds and shouldn'ts we have from the Rule Maker, the more ammunition the Inner Critic has because one of its primary functions is to uphold these rules.

So it is that Jane's Critic attacks her for getting upset with her children and her husband. It criticizes her for being "invaded by thoughts" while she meditates. But, after all, most people get upset with their families from time to time, and learning what to do about this is part of living life fully. Everyone is invaded by thoughts during meditation. Learning how to handle these thoughts is what meditative practice is all about. The voice of the Critic makes each of its pronouncements sound like absolute truth. Who would dare to question its statements?

Arnie has a different kind of Critic. He is the kind of person who is always reacting and telling people how he feels about them. His Rule Maker requires him to be tough, but he has another voice that wants him to be sensitive to people's needs. His Critic attacks him for hurting people and for being insensitive to their feelings and needs. He initially was a shy, introverted youngster, and as he grew up he was very sensitive and quite vulnerable. Since he had to live on the streets of New York, being soft and sensitive did not work for him. It got him beaten up with great regularity, so he had to learn how to be tough and hard. Softness meant pain.

The vulnerability, shyness, and tenderness that operated early in his life was buried and is now unavailable to Arnie. But the Inner Critic plays off this sensitivity. It is afraid that his anger, reactivity, and hardness result in people not liking him, which in fact is often the case. Critics are very resourceful about criticism. Whatever works is good enough. Sometimes, as with Arnie, they use their understanding of our disowned selves to more effectively critique us.

AN INNER CRITIC POTPOURRI OF SELF-IMPROVEMENT

Because there are so many viewpoints in the world of self-improvement, the Critic has a field day. Let us listen to a few of the choice selections that we have taken from Voice Dialogue conversations:

He is not being authentic. (This is a popular one in personal growth circles.)

He didn't say that from his essential being.

She needs to be more open. / She needs to be more reserved.

She is not a very good daughter / sister / friend/ mother.

His body is too rigid. It needs work.

She doesn't have a good personality: it is too outgoing / it isn't outgoing enough / there is too much fear / there is too much vulnerability / he's not real enough / she's too personal / he's too impersonal / she is too much in the transpersonal / her writing is pedestrian.

He (or she) is not in touch with: his feelings / her sexuality / his spirituality / her body / his higher mind / her emotional life / his core.

His energies are off. / Her auric field is not clear.

We could go on for hours listing these comments of the Critic. We have heard each of them hundreds of times during our Voice Dialogue work. What a field day all this is for the therapy profession! What therapist, counselor, or teacher can go hungry with such goings-on? *To teach anything in personal growth work or to study personal growth work without an understanding of the Critic and how it works is going to add to the power and the strength of the Critic!*

As a client or student, too much of what is transmitted in books and workshops and therapy becomes dogma for the Rule Maker/Critic combination. For the teacher or therapist too much gets communicated in a way that lends itself to the interpretation of the Critic. The emphasis of too much therapy and too much personal growth work is on trying to find out what is wrong with people and then fixing them. This fundamental attitude is one of the main reasons why people can come out of extensive personal growth work with Critics that weigh three thousand pounds. So long as therapists and teachers are parental "knowers," Inner Critics will gain weight. Rather than discovering what is wrong, let us discover who we are and how we work. Let us become aware of the amazing system of selves that lives inside us and see how they interact. Then let us learn to have more choice in how to use them. In this way, we are all in the same boat, all fellow explorers, and the Inner Critic does not have the same fuel available to it.

THE CRITIC AS DEBATER

One of the things that makes things additionally difficult is that the Critic is schooled in debate. It can take any side of any question, and often you will hear it take both sides of the same question with the same person. One of the greatest challenges in learning to deal with the Inner Critic is to begin to recognize that the content of what is being said is not important. It is the energy behind it that is central to our understanding. A Critic may say to you, "That really did not work out very well!" You feel depressed and down. You focus on what did not work out and why. That is not the issue. The issue is that someone is hurting you. No matter how good or how well-meant the reaction of the Critic, if it is said with a knife (or choke hold or hit on the head) then the issue is to recognize the energy of the voice and to realize that it is wielding a dangerous weapon against you. You can deal with the details of the content at some other time.

Listen to the following Voice Dialogue conversation with Ellen. She has been talking about her problem with her girlfriend and how she feels very critical of herself with her friends:

FACILITATOR (to Critic): Ellen says that she feels very critical of herself in regard to her friendships. I have to assume that this is you operating inside of her.

CRITIC: Well, of course it's me. She is too aggressive in her relationships. She needs to hang back more, play more hard to get. She's just too open.

FACILITATOR: It sounds as though you're suggesting that she be a little more manipulative with her friends, not let it all hang out there.

CRITIC: No, she can't be manipulative. She has to be there with the other person. I want her to be real and authentic.

FACILITATOR: But you said before that you felt she was too aggressive and too open. Now you say that she should really be there and be authentic. What does that mean to you, to be authentic?

CRITIC: It means being honest and clear without any game playing. She needs to be much stronger. She needs to be able to show her real feelings. She also is too needy. I can't stand her neediness. She needs to be more self-sufficient. I want her to have more friends.

In this brief conversation the Critic has told Ellen, through the facilitator, that she is too aggressive and too open; it wants her to be more honest and authentic; she needs to be stronger; she is too needy; she must be able to express all of her feelings. Aside from all this confused content, there is a more central issue and that is the assaultive nature of the communication. The emotional attack is what we must learn to listen for. This is just a plain, everyday Critic conversation, the type that is going on in our heads constantly. Is it any wonder that aspirin is so widely used? To say that the Inner Critic can give you a headache is a vast understatement.

THE IQ OF THE INNER CRITIC

We have often felt that it would be valuable to give IQ tests to the subpersonalities. How different the results would be! The Inner Critic would probably score two to three times higher than we, ourselves, would score. The Critic is amazingly bright. Its mind works with the swiftness of a high-speed computer. It is able to jump from one area to another, find the weak spots, and defend its arguments and attacks in a way that is quite awesome.

There is no greater testimony to the intelligence of the Critic than the fact that it has remained hidden all these years.

It is not that people are unaware of being critical of themselves. You will hear people say all the time, "I'm very critical of myself about this or that." However, it is not "I" who is critical of me, it is my Critic who is critical of me. That is the step we must learn to take. Every time we become aware that we are critical of ourselves, we must take the next step. We must be smarter and more aware than the Critic. We must learn to step back into our Aware Ego and say, "That is not me who is critical of myself. That is my old, tried-and-true friend, the Inner Critic. He (or she or it) is the one who is criticizing me. He must be feeling vulnerable or anxious about something. I shall have to talk to him and find out what he is upset about. Otherwise he will stay at me all day." In this way we support the process of separation from the Critic, we help to alleviate the anxiety of the Critic, and gradually we help transform the Critic into a part of our creative and discerning mind that can operate under our control.

◆ WHAT IS YOUR CRITIC'S AGENDA FOR YOU?

1. How many books do you have in your bedroom waiting to be read? What does your Critic say to you about the fact that you have not read those books?

2. What does your Critic say to you about the way that you eat? How does it want you to improve your health?

3. What are some other areas in which your Critic feels that you should do better? Consider physical, mental, emotional, and spiritual improvement.

4. To whom does your Critic compare you? Who can do it (whatever *it* is) better? Who is more evolved than you are?

Chapter Six

Critic Attacks and How to Deal with Them

It is our job to learn to see underneath these attacks and to discover the very soft, tender, and terrified core that lies beneath the tough, aggressive, and attacking bravado of our Critic friend.

The Inner Critic is active for varying amounts of time in each of us. For more people than you could possibly imagine, it is practically a full-time operation. In other instances it plays a lesser role. In our experience, it is operating to some degree in everyone. Some people are not aware of their Inner Critic because, instead of criticizing themselves, they spend their time judging other people. However, if life deals them a blow that breaks their power, such as a divorce or illness, the Critic is right there doing its job.

Many times during the day we are subject to what we call "Critic Attacks." In these special moments the Inner Critic comes to the fore in full glory and blasts us with everything that it has. These are the times when we feel truly dreadful about ourselves. Often outside influences lead to these kinds of attacks, though this is not always the case. We would like to discuss some of the things that happen in our lives that can lead us to be more vulnerable and thus more susceptible to the attack of the Inner Critic.

JUDGMENTS

One of the most basic outer events that leads to a Critic Attack is having another person criticize or judge us. This outer criticism arouses our Inner Critic, who becomes anxious. Being criticized makes us feel very vulnerable. No one likes to be criticized. A sense of shame and guilt and a threat to self-esteem arise in such an experience. In response to this vulnerability, our Inner Critic goes into action. After all, one of its basic jobs since early childhood was to protect us from criticism by criticizing us first!

Any of the important (or even unimportant) people in our lives can judge us. Advertisements telling us to look young, be thin, be healthy, be joyous can all be interpreted as judgments. With so many available judges on the outer level, it is often difficult to realize that there is also a Critic on the inner level. Learning to deal with the outer judges can be a big help in shifting the Inner Critic in some situations, but it is just as often the case that one solves the problem of an outer judge and the Inner Critic remains stronger and perhaps even more impregnable than ever. This frequently happens when people break from very judgmental parents. By getting out of the house and trying not to have anything to do with such a parent, they think that the problem of judgment is solved. Not so at all! On an inner level the judgmental voice is more powerful than ever and, in many cases, even more effective because they do not know that it exists.

We also see this when people break from a strict religious upbringing that is perceived as too judgmental. They revolt against the narrowness and judgmental nature of a fundamentalist belief structure and then adopt a totally different value system that is quite opposite to the original one. Such a person will go through life hating fundamentalists and fundamentalist doctrines and never realize that a powerful Fundamentalist Self has allied with the Critic and continues to live deep within, echoing these early teachings.

When someone in our environment criticizes us, we are fighting a difficult battle. We have the person outside of us to deal with, and we have the person inside us, who is invisible and unknown to us, to deal with as well. We may feel the pain of the outer criticism, but we will not be able to find the focus of the pain and anguish caused by our inner adversary because it is invisible. Generally we just feel depressed, anxious, vaguely upset, headachy, or without energy. Once the cloak of invisibility of the Inner Critic is lifted, then our dealings with the judges of the outer world can change very much in our favor. Imagine dealing with an adversary standing in front of you when an invisible man is standing behind you hitting you on the head and choking you at the same time!

The core of the outer judgments goes something like this: "The trouble with you is . . . !" This is the lament and litany of the judges of the world. It is fixed in our minds like a religious mantra. The trouble with you is . . . ! The trouble with you is. . . ! The trouble with you is . . . ! For many people it starts in early childhood and never stops for a moment throughout the rest of their lives. If we grow up with this litany on the outside, then the Inner Critic develops a corresponding music. Sung to whatever melody it chooses, the Inner Critic's refrain is always the same as the outer judgments: The trouble with you is. . . . The trouble with you is. . . . The trouble with you is. . . . At some level this is always part of the core feeling of a Critic Attack.

Not all judgments toward us are overt, however. We receive a great deal of negativity from our environment in ways that are much more subtle. For example, John comes home from work, and after he gets settled in for a few minutes he asks his wife, "Did you get a chance to pick up my shirts today?" It sounds like an innocent question, but so often in relationships these kinds of questions have a hidden agenda. What he is feeling, underneath the question, is the real issue. Many people have a difficult time expressing their real feelings to each other. Every unspoken feeling has the possibility of becoming a judgment directed toward the other person. A direct reaction may sting, but it at least lets us know something of the reality of the person who is expressing the feeling. Silent judgments do their work without our knowledge.

Mary feels guilty when John asks about his shirts. She becomes apologetic and contrite. She is responding like a daughter to an unconscious judgment underlying John's question. Her Critic is agreeing with his silent judgment and attacking her from within. However, what John is really feeling underneath is that she is not paying enough attention to him, that she is neglecting his needs, that she spends too much time with the children and with her friends. He knows nothing of these feelings or of his vulnerability in general. The judgmental voice in him is his refuge so that he does not have to feel hurt by her. The general rule might be expressed this way: *Whenever someone is not in touch with his or her vulnerability in relationship to another person, one may expect a judgment, silent or spoken, as a way of dealing with the situation.* Unconscious vulnerability is a very dangerous commodity for this reason.

Sam and Helen are having dinner at a restaurant. It is a rather elegant restaurant and Helen feels vulnerable here because she feels some inadequacy about her physical appearance. She is not, however, aware of her own discomfort. She starts to feel quite judgmental about the way that Sam is eating. She looks at him and thinks that he is sloppy and without grace. She is very concerned with what the other people who are watching might think of his manners. For his part, Sam starts to eat too fast and to spill his food and to splatter food on his shirt. He begins to feel like a first-class slob, and his Inner Critic goes into action letting him know just exactly what a slob he really is. Not a word has been spoken between them, but she has now gone into a full Judgmental Self and he is in the midst of a first-class Critic Attack. Such are the ways of silent judgment.

STRESS

Any condition of stress is a flash point for the Inner Critic. Here again the Inner Critic responds to vulnerability. It is always playing off our vulnerability because, as we have seen, it was born to protect it. Stress always leaves us more vulnerable if we have not learned how to handle it properly.

Stress is often related to a condition of being over-tired or fatigued. Fatigue, too, makes us more vulnerable than usual. Stress and fatigue tend to diminish the coping ability of the stronger sides of our personality. Whenever our basic coping mechanisms are not working properly, we are more vulnerable and the Inner Critic is likely to attack us for not "being together" or not being strong enough or not having control of a situation or being too unfocused or ten thousand other descriptive phrases that it knows so well how to use. Underneath all this, of course, is its basic panic that we are not safe in the world and that we cannot handle life. Since there is much insecurity in life and much stress, the Inner Critic has an available entry point much of the time.

DISOWNED SELVES

Another time the Critic attacks is when one of our disowned selves breaks out in some social or business situation. The Inner Critic is terribly afraid that we will look foolish or behave shamefully. In this sense it behaves exactly like a parent, which, in effect, it is. Disowned selves are those parts of us that are not allowed to come out because our main ways of being in the world simply will not permit it. So, for example, the part of us that requires control does not want a more spontaneous or free spirit to emerge in us because this might be dangerous. We might do something that would make us look foolish or cause us real embarrassment or shame. The Inner Critic remembers the pain of these kinds of feelings that occurred so often in the growing-up process and does not want this repeated.

Let us say that Alice goes to a party and has a few drinks. Soon her Spontaneous Self comes out and she starts cutting up and singing and flirting and having a lot of fun. The next morning, perhaps 2:00 or 4:00 A.M., her Critic starts to attack. This is a favorite time for the Inner Critic because at this hour of the morning we tend to be in a fairly vulnerable position and our usual defenses are not available to us. Critics love to dredge up what we did wrong the night before, the day before, the week before, the month before, even ten years before. Its memory is unbelievable. Thus it happens that the disowned self had its way with Alice the night before, but the Inner Critic has its way with her now! It is going to do everything it can to restore the proper control so that things will be safe again. The physical hangover from too much drinking is nothing compared to the psychological hangover that comes from such Critic Attacks, especially the early morning variety.

Often people who live with strong control will drink or use drugs to get rid of the control. Like Alice, they are then free to act out their disowned selves. But the Inner Critics gain weight whenever this happens, and they have a tendency to come soaring back like birds of prey once the control side returns to power.

UNFAMILIAR SITUATIONS

Being in any kind of unfamiliar situation is another thing that tends to activate the Critic. Here, again, the basic issue is vulnerability. Traveling to unknown places, having a new child, entering into a new job or a new program of some kind—each of these can make us more vulnerable. The primary ways of behaving in the world are threatened because we are in an unknown place. The moment we feel vulnerable and cannot deal with or are not aware of this vulnerability, then the Critic is ready to move in.

WHEN WE ARE AT THE CENTER OF ATTENTION

The Inner Critic is waiting to pounce on us any time we do something that makes us the center of attention. Performance and evaluation are the keys here. Being evaluated can make us more vulnerable and thus more sensitive to a Critic invasion. If we consider for a moment the way our school system operates, we get a chance to see how the Inner Critic can become so powerful. From our earliest years, we are constantly being graded for our behavior, effort, learning ability, and knowledge. We are constantly being judged and criticized by the very nature of the educational process that evaluates everything that we do. This alone can nourish and fatten an Inner Critic to heavy-weight proportions.

ADVERSE FORTUNE

Adverse fortune is also likely to bring on Critic Attacks. Examples of this might be the loss of a job, failing a class, or being left (abandoned) by a friend or partner. Economic instability is an important factor here. Whenever we are experiencing economic difficulties, we are much more likely to feel the power of the Critic. Each of these examples of adverse fortune represents a powerful threat, which activates our vulnerability and invites in the Inner Critic, who forever lives in terror of abandonment and not being able to make it in the world. The more terrorized it feels, the more vicious will be its attack on us.

It is our job to learn to see underneath these attacks and to discover the very soft, tender, and terrified core that lies beneath the tough, aggressive, and attacking bravado of our Critic friend. *Killer rage and vulnerability are two sides of a coin, whether that rage be directed outwardly or inwardly.* As we have said before and we will say again, disowned vulnerability makes for a very dangerous playmate!

DO CERTAIN PEOPLE IN YOUR LIFE TRIGGER
CRITIC ATTACKS?

Is there someone in your life who consistently brings on Critic Attacks in you? If so, something in this relationship is not working properly for you. Perhaps the other person is carrying one of your disowned selves. When you overvalue another person so that just being with that person makes you feel inferior, it is often a sign that the other carries a disowned self. To check this out, do the second part of the disowned self exercise at the end of Chapter 1. You might find that this other person carries a self that you have disowned over the years.

For example, whenever Eleanor is with Alicia, a woman who is always elegantly attired, Eleanor begins to feel like a slob. Her Critic is saying something like, "You look pretty frumpy next to her. Nobody is going to notice you, and if they do, they'll see how much better she looks." Soon Eleanor's Critic is moving into other areas of her life and a full-scale Critic Attack is under way.

Now, Eleanor is a woman whose primary self values sobriety, simplicity, and hard work. This self believes that paying attention to the way she looks would be wasteful and in decidedly poor taste. Eleanor's primary self would disapprove of any time or money spent on what it would consider superficial and useless activities. Eleanor, therefore, has no choice about her appearance. It is her primary self that makes these decisions for her, and it is her Critic who supports these decisions. Therefore, Eleanor's Critic Attacks are signaling Eleanor that she is ignoring an entire aspect of her own personality, the part of her that, like Alicia, would simply love to spend time on her appearance.

Perhaps this person who usually triggers Critic Attacks in you has a primary self that characteristically puts down other people and must always feel superior to them. Or perhaps this person reminds you of your parents or of a powerful sibling and this memory re-activates your Critic's anxiety for your safety. As you think about this, you can use this person as a teacher to help you to learn more about yourself. Of course, after seeing the pattern of Critic Attacks, you may wish to avoid a certain kind of contact with this person.

If someone in your life consistently triggers Critic Attacks, it is time for you to discover what this kind of relationship is all about, whether through your own personal work or with the help of a psychotherapist. There is no need to remain in the state of misery that this kind of relationship creates.

DEALING WITH CRITIC ATTACKS

At the end of this chapter, we have included some suggestions about noting the times and places of your own Critic Attacks. In looking over these times and places, you may discover interesting patterns. Often attacks occur when people are hungry, tired, or lonesome. If so, it is a good idea to start to pay attention to your eating and sleeping patterns. You might also pay attention to your social contacts to be sure that you spend enough time with others so that you are not lonely. Some kinds of food bring on Critic Attacks. We have known people who are particularly susceptible to attacks after eating sugar or consuming caffeine in one form or another. Sometimes Critic Attacks result from the food itself. Sometimes they can be a function of the New Age Critic telling us that sugar and caffeine are bad for us. Some people get Critic Attacks after drinking just because of the effect of the alcohol itself. Each of us is different, and you might use your Critic Attacks to get an idea of what it is that you are doing that really does not agree with you.

You might find that you are particularly susceptible at certain times of the day or night. Critics simply love to attack in the wee hours of the morning. If you lie in bed and allow your Inner Critic to tell you that you are an incurable insomniac and to review the mistakes of your life for you, you are in deep trouble! If you know how to meditate or if you pray, this is a good time to do so. If you have other relaxation techniques, this is a good time to use them. If you cannot calm yourself and get back to sleep, our suggestion is to get out of bed and do something. Doing something, anything, is better than passively lying in bed as victim and prey to the Inner Critic.

Many people find that personal writing, either some form of journal writing or writing down dreams (telling them as stories or actually working with them), is best. If this does not appeal to you, do something pleasant or distracting, like reading a book, having a glass of warm milk or herbal tea, or listening to some favorite soothing music. These techniques can often calm the Critic's anxiety and allow you to feel less vulnerable.

If you are a more active or extraverted type, get some work done. After all, you are awake anyway and your brain is fully functioning. You might even take this opportunity to tackle some unattractive job that you have been putting off. Then, not only do you soften the Critic Attack, but you literally take care of the Critic's underlying anxiety by getting some unfinished work done!

When you recognize an incipient Critic Attack, say to yourself, "I smell a Critic Attack coming on and I'm going to do something about it." Then, as we have said before, do something, anything, other than lie there passively and let it happen.

If your Critic attacks are stress related, think about the stresses in your life and what you might be able to do about them. This might mean restructuring your schedule or re-arranging your priorities. It might also mean that it is time for you to finish some particular task that remains undone and that is currently costing you more energy not to do than it would cost you to do it.

YOUR INNER CRITIC AND THE STRESS IN YOUR LIFE

Not only does your Inner Critic respond to the stresses in your life, but it also introduces its own stresses in addition to those already present. It is not just the content of its criticisms and the difficulty (or impossibility) of its goals, but the constant vicious attack of the Inner Critic—the relentless, heartless, stress-inducing pressure that it exerts—that damages you.

Now you have the opportunity to determine your Critic's expectations of you. You already know some of its agenda for self-improvement from your responses to the exercises at the end of chapter 5. Is it possible that you overlooked anything else that needs improvement? If so, add it to this list of things you should do now. Look at this agenda for self-improvement and realize that it was set by your Inner Critic with the help of your primary selves. It can be altered. *Now separate from the requirements of your Inner Critic, remember that you will never satisfy it, and reevaluate this agenda.* There may be parts of this agenda that you, yourself, think are important, and there may be others that seem completely unnecessary or even inappropriate for you to worry about. If you wish, you might do this reevaluation with your small group, with individuals that you trust, or with a therapist or teacher who will help you to evolve a more realistic and appropriate set of expectations for yourself. This kind of periodic reevaluation should help you to reduce the stress that your Inner Critic introduces into your life.

THE FREEDOM TO BE ORDINARY

If we could encourage one major step in this reevaluation of your Inner Critic's agenda, it would be: give yourself permission to be ordinary! The need to be special adds immeasurably to the stress in your life. We do not mean that you should become careless or satisfied with mediocrity. What we do mean is that you should get off the runaway Special Express train and live your life with fewer demands for extraordinary achievement. *When you are no longer focused upon amazing others or surpassing them, you have much more energy available to do your best.* You are no longer spending half your time looking over your shoulder at what others are doing or comparing yourself to them.

You do not have to do this all at once. Reevaluating your Inner Critic's agenda is an ongoing process, and each of us needs to work on it on a continuing basis. Each time that you do this re-evaluation, you are taking away the authority of the Inner Critic (and your primary selves) and are assuming the authority and responsibility for directing your life yourself.

♦ WHEN AND WHERE DOES YOUR CRITIC ATTACK?

Let us look at your own special Critic Attacks, those times when your Inner Critic runs amok and there seems to be nothing that you can do to stop it.

1. Some people always leave us feeling bad about ourselves. Who are the people in your life who consistently bring on Critic Attacks in you? Once you have thought of someone, consider the following questions:

   a. Close your eyes and visualize the last time you were to-gether or the last time that you spoke with each other. What exactly did he or she do or say that made you feel bad? (It usually is a direct or implied judgment or a comparison of some kind.) Try to recall this as specifically as you can.

   b. What was your response? Can you picture or remember what happened?

   c. Can you make the connection between the Critic Attack and what was said to you?

   d. Can you see situations where this happens with other people?

2. Over the next three days, pay careful attention to your pattern of Critic Attacks. After they pass and you are feeling somewhat better, try to understand what caused them. Do they happen at a particular time of day or with a particular person? Were you criticized? Were you under stress? Did your husband say something to you? Were you particularly hungry or tired? Examine what happened in the light of the examples that we have given in this chapter.

3. At some time when you are not in the middle of a Critic Attack, think about your own pattern of attacks and, using the information and suggestions in this chapter, see if you can begin to figure out ways of dealing with them. Pretend that you are giving advice to someone else about how to deal with the situations that leave you open to attacks. If at any point you feel your Critic taking over, wait a while and come back to this work at another time, either alone or with someone else.

Chapter Seven

The Inner Critic's Role in Shame, Depression, and Low Self-Esteem

We personally feel that many of the common psychological problems in this current era are due to the virulence of the Inner Critic. We live in a culture and at a time in history when being truly human is not enough; we must all be more and better. For the most part, we are not encouraged to look at ourselves objectively, take stock of what we see, and realistically set about living our lives in harmony with the deepest needs of our innermost being. Instead, we must continually improve upon ourselves. This provides fertile ground for the growth of the Inner Critic.

Do you suffer from low self-esteem? Most of us do.

The concept of low self-esteem has been around for ages. It is like a virus that everyone seems to catch from time to time; we all recognize it and understand what it is about. Basically, you just do not feel good about yourself. You do not like who you are. You do not feel particularly worthy. You have trouble standing up for yourself, asserting yourself, or thinking that anyone wants to have anything to do with you either professionally or personally. Some people suffer chronically, some occasionally, and some cover the signs of low self-esteem by performing amazing feats at the urging of their Pushers and Perfectionists, fooling themselves and many onlookers into thinking that they must feel just marvelous about themselves.

Low self-esteem has been one of the most popularized forms of psychological discomfort, and well it might be because it is so prevalent. Many articles have been written in the popular press about how to recognize its symptoms and how to deal with it. One of the problems that this introduces is that once you know you have low self-esteem, you begin to feel ashamed that you do, and this just adds to your feeling inferior.

People can feel bad about themselves for many reasons, but we suspect that a major factor in this malaise known as low self-esteem is the undercover activity of the Inner Critic. If someone is constantly telling you what is wrong with you and if you believe what he says, how can you possibly feel good about yourself?

WHY CAN'T I FEEL SUCCESSFUL?

You cannot feel successful because your Inner Critic will not let you! It is often as simple as that. No matter what you do, it is not quite enough. The Critic with its superior intelligence, its superhuman sensing devices, and its access to the secret files of your mistakes or failures, will just not let you feel successful.

How can you feel successful when someone is constantly reminding you of your shortcomings, of what you did wrong or what you probably will do wrong? Let us listen to some of the things your Critic might say when you actually do reach a goal.

Yes, indeed, you do well at work, but it's at the expense of a personal life.

You have your work and your personal life under control, but your body is a mess or your relationship with your parents is still unresolved.

It took you longer than anyone else to get where you are.

They don't know the mistakes you made before you reached this goal.

It doesn't matter, all your friends have done equally well or better.

You may be successful, but you still don't have real wealth.

Yes, you have money, but you have no real career or
profession.

Nobody really cares.

You fooled everybody. You didn't really do that well.
(This is usually accompanied by a list of what is still
wrong or missing or what you had better do in the future to follow up.)

Your brother (sister, father, mother, friend, associate)
would have done it better (or faster).

Your Inner Critic, in its attempt to keep you from disap-
pointment or shame, will not allow you to feel good about what
you have accomplished. It is often afraid that if you feel good,
someone will take that feeling away from you. It is better not
to feel good; then you will not be disappointed. Sometimes your
Inner Critic fears the envy of others or their possible criticism, so
it tries to prepare you for this in advance by criticizing you first.

Sometimes, the Inner Critic is genuinely concerned with the
sin of pride. Some critics have a deeply religious base and they
fear that you will become too proud. It is their job to keep you
humble and thankful, to remind you of your place, and to guard
against inflation and self-aggrandizement. It can be quite cruel as
it does this.

SHAME

The brilliant work of John Bradshaw has given us an entirely
new understanding of one of our culture's most prevalent and
painful psychological problems. He has introduced the concept
of toxic shame, the "shame that binds you," and has shown how
deeply and destructively it affects lives. As he says in *Healing the
Shame That Binds You*:

> To be shame bound means that whenever you feel any feeling,
> any need or any drive, you immediately feel ashamed. The dy-
> namic core of your life is grounded in your feelings, your needs
> and your drives. When these are bound by shame, you are
> shamed to the core.

He goes on to show how this shame destroys us and how it can be the root cause for all kinds of addictive and abusive behavior. He shows how it operates in codependency, in narcissistic and borderline personality disorders, and in depression. He explains how it is indicative of spiritual bankruptcy.

We would like to ask the question, "Who is it that shames you?" For us, of course, the answer is The Inner Critic. It is your Critic who feels you are rotten to the core. It is your Critic who feels you must never let anyone know who or what you are because you are a mistake; you are a flawed, an evil, possibly even a dangerous, creature. It is your Critic who fears that others will find you disgusting or possibly horrifying and that they will hurt or reject you.

Much as your parents did before, your Critic shames you so that you will change your behavior (even if you cannot change your "rotten core"). It hopes, as your parents did before it, that if you do disguise who you are and how you feel, then perhaps, just perhaps, you will be more acceptable to others.

In cases of toxic shame, your Inner Critic's deepest fear is that you are basically rotten and flawed, that you are a mistake, and that there is nothing good within you. It works tirelessly to see who you are and then to change you. Since it must make you into something other than what you are, it moves you ever farther away from your own natural feelings, needs, and desires. It tries to get you to be someone who it imagines will be acceptable to others.

If your Critic is constantly leveling major attacks upon your very being; if it sees everything about you as flawed; and if you have lost touch with the fact that you are, indeed, a child of the universe, then you are living in shame. You feel you do not deserve to be and you must apologize for your very existence. You must do whatever you can to make life bearable. Unfortunately, many of the things that you do to make life bearable (such as addictive, codependent, or antisocial behavior) prove just how bad you are, the Critic panics and intensifies its attacks, you feel even more ashamed, and the cycle continues.

THE SPECIAL ADVANTAGE OF THE INNER CRITIC

We have alluded to the special advantage of the Inner Critic, but this is such an important point that we would like to mention it again. The advantage of the Inner Critic is just that—it is inner! It knows you from the inside, and, in addition, it is generally invisible.

It knows all the parts of your personality that you are trying to hide from other people, for whatever reasons you may have. It knows about the parts of you that you feel are not nice and that you feel ashamed about. If you look self-assured, it knows that you feel nervous inside. If you are kind and generous, it knows that sometimes you feel selfish. If you finish a task, it knows what you have left undone. It knows all the mean, uncharitable, cruel feelings that you have inside. It knows about your sexual fantasies. It knows when you are needy and vulnerable even though you might be able to hide this from others.

Your Inner Critic knows about all your deepest, darkest secrets, the ones that you really want to hide. And, using this classified information, it criticizes you unmercifully.

DANGER—DEPRESSION AHEAD!

As the Inner Critic gains leverage, it can tilt us into a rather serious depression. As its power increases, we may even begin to feel that life is just too much trouble. Why bother to get up in the morning? Why bother to dress? Why bother to go out working or even looking for a job? After all, why try to do anything when you know that nothing will ever be good enough? The next step in all this is a feeling of paralysis, and from this place it is very easy to feel that life is no longer worth living.

It is apparent by now that if we look beneath most of our feelings of discomfort about ourselves, we can usually find our old pal, the Inner Critic, at work examining us, evaluating us, finding us inferior, and generally undermining the very foundations of our self-worth. As we have said before, once we hear the voice of this Critic as it broadcasts on station KRAZY, we no longer have to listen to what it is telling us but instead can direct our energies and our problem-solving skills toward the source of the discomfort, the Inner Critic itself.

Chapter Eight

The Critic as Abuser of the Inner Child

As difficult as it is to escape an outer abuser, it is even more diffi-cult to escape one who lives within. The Inner Critic's abuse oc-curs in the privacy of your own mind, and the Inner Child is devastated when nobody else can see or hear or help.

One specific aspect of the Inner Critic's activities is particularly interesting, and that is its role in the cycle of child abuse. It is well known that adults who were abused as children are likely, in turn, to abuse their own children. In a similar fashion, the Inner Critic echoes the criticism or abuse of the outer parent and continues the cycle through the abuse of the Inner Child.

INTRODUCING THE VULNERABLE CHILD

The Inner Child, which includes the Vulnerable Child that we spoke of in chapter 1, has been receiving a great deal of attention recently. We are very glad that it has, because for a long time we have felt that the Inner Child, especially in its vulnerable as-pect, is one of the most important players in our inner cast of characters.

Who is this Vulnerable Child? It is the vulnerable little crea-ture we all were when we were first born. This child was and is exquisitely sensitive. It responds to energies rather than to words. It feels what is going on around it in the world at large, and it does not try to make sense out of it. It feels everything that is going on inside of us as well. In this way, it is tuned in to all the subtleties of our emotional interactions, both the outer interactions with people on the outside and the inner ones with our very own selves.

This Inner Child has many aspects. In addition to the Vulnerable Child, who carries our deepest feelings, sensitivities, and vulnerabilities, other aspects of the Inner Child carry major portions of our spontaneity, shyness, neediness, fears, joy, magic, our ability to be unselfconscious, our playfulness, and our adventurousness. The Inner Child can be extremely angry with us or with others when we neglect or mistreat it.

It is the Vulnerable Child who is one of the major players in making intimacy possible in relationship. We speak about this in our book *Embracing Each Other.* When the Vulnerable Child is present in relationship you can actually feel it. There is an almost palpable warmth between you and others and the air feels full between you. When this Child is not there, you feel empty and alone.

This Inner Child, and all its aspects, is usually buried pretty early in our growing-up process. The world is not safe for someone of its sensitivities, so it goes underground and the other selves take over in order to run our lives as successfully and efficiently as they can. These are the primary selves we talked about in chapter 1. But just because we cannot see it does not mean that the Child is no longer there. It is present always, hiding somewhere in the back of the closet, up in its treehouse, or deep in a cave. From its hiding place it sees, hears, and feels, but we are not aware that this is happening.

THE CRITIC IS A CRUEL AND ABUSIVE PARENT

What happens to this exquisitely sensitive child when your Inner Critic is operating? It gets abused. Badly! This abuse can range from mild to vicious, depending upon the circumstances of your upbringing. But the abuse is always present to some degree.

Your Inner Critic was born to protect your Inner Child and to keep it from harm. Its role was to help you fit in, to conform to the world around you. No matter how gently this is done, the message is clear: your Child's natural behavior is unacceptable, and something is wrong with its natural instincts. Because of the Vulnerable Child's acute sensitivity, this criticism is very painful.

Now let us think about what happens when your parents have actually been insensitive or, worse yet, abusive. The Critic models itself on the outer authorities, so, in this case, it will model itself on your abusive parents. If your parents abuse you, your Critic will abuse you in a similar fashion. If your parents live shame-based lives, they will shame you and your Critic, in turn, will pick up their messages and shame you. And the Inner Critic usually increases the intensity of the abuse just to be sure that you will be adequately protected and prepared for what might come in from the outside.

Thus, in our conversations with the Inner Critic, we often hear the echoes of the abusive parents:

He's an idiot.

She's a bother and a pest. Even her mother wished she'd
    go away.

She's a whore.

I wish he had never been born. There's something
    wrong that I can't seem to beat out of him.

She's nothing but trouble.

He's useless.

Success is out of the question. Nobody in this family suc-
    ceeds.

He'll never amount to anything.

There's only one thing she's good for . . .

She's ugly and nothing will ever help.

Nobody ever really liked her.

He's disgusting.

She's too bossy.

If he didn't get beaten, he would do terrible things.

If nobody disciplined her, she'd bring shame to the
    family.

Nobody could love a person like that! Even her mother
  told her that.

He doesn't deserve any better.

People have to force themselves to be nice to him.

At some point, usually fairly early in the developmental
process, the abusive Inner Critic has grown beyond its original
boundaries and takes on an uncontrollable life of its own. It
forgets its original purpose, which was to protect you from the
outer abuse, and it just abuses you because that is what it does. It
knows that you are bad and that you deserve all the vicious
comments that it is making. Worse yet, it is likely to be con-
vinced that there is something very wrong with you, that you
are basically evil or flawed, and that its criticisms are therefore
justified. In addition to all this, it sounds infallible, as we dis-
cussed in chapter 3.

Now you have within you an abuser, and a major part of
you that is being battered by its endless, and seemingly justified, abuse is your Inner Child. This creates intense psychic pain.
Sometimes the Inner Critic will arrange for actual physical abuse
to be added to this psychological abuse. In these cases, the Inner
Critic is actually unable to rest until some punishment has been
received; some actual physical suffering or great emotional pain
is required. Then the Critic is relieved, it knows that it has done
its job, and it knows peace for a short while.

THE DIFFICULTY IN ESCAPING THE ABUSER

As difficult as it is to escape from an outer abuser, it is even more
difficult to escape the one who lives within. The Inner Critic's
abuse occurs in the privacy of your own mind, and the Child (or
any other self) is hurt when nobody else can see or hear. The
picture is a very touching one; it is as though your Inner Child
is locked away with your Inner Critic and there is no way in
which you or anyone else can rescue it.

Many of you who have been abused work hard to escape the
outer abuser but then cannot escape the abuser within. We feel

that working with the Inner Critic is extremely important. When you are unable to separate from an abusive Inner Critic, you are kept in victim status. With the Critic criticizing you, you feel flawed, as though you deserve the worst that the world has to offer. You cannot protect yourself. This makes you a victim, fully available to anyone on the outside who would hurt you. As a victim, you will draw abusers to you, and you will accept their abuse.

There is an amazing irony about this inner abuse. All of this can be going on inside of you and you do not even know about it. All you know is that you feel pretty rotten about yourself and you seem to keep getting into hurtful situations. Thus, the abuse of your Inner Child is a secret even from you and if you do not see it you cannot do anything about it. One thing we can say for sure. *If you keep drawing abusive people into your life, you may be sure that the Inner Critic is operating in you in an abusive way.*

THE SECRECY OF THE INNER CRITIC

There is an interesting catch-22 in the way that the Inner Critic operates. In order for you to work with your Inner Critic, you must expose it to someone on the outside, much as the victim of child abuse must bring outside attention to the abuse before anything can be done about it.

If you are aware of your Inner Critic's voice, the Critic itself will tell you that it would be simply dreadful for you to let anyone know about it. After all, if you tell others about it, they will listen to its complaints and then they will see things wrong with you that they might not otherwise have noticed. So you try to keep it a secret so that nobody will ever hear the terrible things that it knows about you. After all, it is probably right!

The more that you think of the things the Critic has to say, the more embarrassed you get and the less likely you are going to want to expose it—and your deepest, darkest shortcomings—to the world.

If this need for secrecy blocks you, then the entire cycle of (inner) child abuse remains out of reach. You cannot let others hear your Critic so that they might help you. You cannot gain access to your Aware Ego, which might be able to see things differently and would most certainly have other tools at its disposal. You are left alone with your shameful secrets, which grow ever more fetid in the dark closets of your psyche, and a Critic who keeps reminding you how truly disgusting they are.

A CONVERSATION WITH THE INNER CHILD AFTER A CRUEL CRITIC HAS BEEN TALKING

Let us hear how the Inner Child feels after it has been listening to an Inner Critic. The facilitator had been talking to Anna's Inner Critic for quite some time. This Critic sounded a lot like Anna's mother who was abusive to her when she was young. Suddenly Anna burst into tears. The facilitator realized that the Inner Child, who had been listening to all this abuse, had broken through. She asked Anna to move over and then began to talk to the Inner Child as follows:

FACILITATOR: You were listening, weren't you?

CHILD (sobbing): Did you hear what she said? I can't stand it anymore. I just can't stand it. Sometimes I just want to stay in bed and never get up. It's awful. It's just not worth it.

FACILITATOR: What's awful?

CHILD: I'm so alone. So alone! So alone! (She sobs more.) I never get to feel okay about anything. I'm always scared. She (meaning the Critic) is always screaming and screaming at me. Whatever I do, it's no good. No matter what I look like, I'm ugly. It's no use! I can't do anything right. I'm stupid and clumsy and nobody ever helps me. My mom really doesn't like me either. She used to punish me a lot. She didn't want me to play with other kids. She said I was bad and that people didn't like me and that's true. I never had any friends.

FACILITATOR: It's dreadful to be so alone.

CHILD: You bet. I don't have a single person I can turn to. I'm really afraid. Every time I want to make a friend, she (the Critic) tells me they won't like me anyway once they get to know me, because I'm not nice, so I don't even want to try. Besides, nobody would really want me for a friend. I think there's something wrong with me. She says there is. And so if people ever really saw me, they'd run away. Everybody has. (Sighing) I'm just a pest and people don't like me. Don't you think I'm a pest? I'd better be quiet now.

This conversation gives a picture of what happens to the Inner Child after years of abuse. It is alone and afraid. It thinks that there is something wrong with it. It is terrified that if it speaks out, it will be rejected. Although it desperately needs others, it cannot reach out.

BREAKING THE CYCLE OF CHILD ABUSE

Once you become aware of the Inner Critic as a child abuser, you can move in and treat it in much the same way that you break into the outer cycle of child abuse. The Inner Critic learned how to parent you by listening to your own parents. If they were abusive, it repeats their abuse "for your own good." It acts just like a real parent who abuses the child because the parent, herself or himself, has been the victim of abuse.

The key to breaking the Inner Critic's cycle of abuse is to separate from the Critic's voice. As you separate from your Inner Critic, you will be able to take over the role of parent to your own Inner Child. Up until now, the Inner Critic has been the parent to the Inner Child; it has been an abusive parent because that is the only way it knew how to behave. Oddly enough, you can become a parent to the Inner Critic as well because you are in a position to deal with the underlying anxiety of the Inner Critic and to stop the Critic from its endless abusive chatter. You will be surprised to find that you have a wide range of knowledge and can make choices. The Inner Critic knows of only one way to cope with life—it knows how to criticize and how to abuse. (For more on learning to parent the Inner Critic, see chapter 17.)

When we work with the Critic as an inner abuser we have a way in which to enter into the outer cycle of abuse as well. Until you separate from the abusive Inner Critic and are no longer dominated by it, you will be kept a victim to everyone around you. As a victim you will draw abusers to you. As a victim you may actually induce the abuser in almost anyone that you meet, even in people who are not normally abusive. You will be unable to protect yourself from their abuse because your Critic will be telling you that you deserve all that you get. Thus, you will forever carry a "fifth column" within yourself, someone who will cooperate with the enemy and betray you to him (or her). As you become more aware of this, you gradually can learn how to silence your Inner Critic and no longer be a victim to the abusers of the world.

Chapter Nine

The Critic as Killer
Disowning Our Instinctual Energy

Because of the socialization process that most of us go through, it is often the case that powerful feelings, emotions, and instinctual energies in general are blocked from moving out into the world. What happens then is that instead of providing us with power in the world, these energies turn sour, begin to fester, and over time become more and more potent and negative inside of us. Ultimately, this disowned mass of instinctuality becomes a killer energy that spills over onto another track, the Inner Critic track, and comes back at us. Thus the Inner Critic is infused with all the power and rage of these disowned instinctual energies.

We have used humor in describing the Inner Critic because we have found that humor is one of the best ways to separate from the Critics of the world. The fact is, however, that the way the Critic affects people's lives is anything but funny. It can effectively paralyze us through the deep sense of depression and feelings of unworthiness that it brings to us. In the case of the Killer Critic, this paralysis can become very extreme and can contribute to suicidal feelings and actual suicides.

WHAT IS A KILLER CRITIC?

Critics vary in how powerful they are. We often refer to them jokingly as lightweight, middleweight, or heavyweight. A good heavyweight Critic starts to move into the two-thousand-pound range and can go much higher than that. To be quite honest, we have not seen very many lightweights. At some point in the heavyweight category the quality of the Inner Critic shifts and one must work differently. One cannot be humorous in relationship to it. One cannot talk to it about the underlying vulnerability or anxiety. Heavyweight Critics just hate us. They want us dead.

These Critics must be treated with the utmost respect. There are good reasons why they are as angry and vicious as they are. It takes longer to find out why they hate so deeply, and it requires a great deal of patience, strength, and skill on the part of the facilitator. Listen to the following Voice Dialogue conversation with Jean, a woman in her thirties who was the adult child of an alcoholic parent and who had been sexually abused by her father from the ages of six through nine.

FACILITATOR (to Critic): You seem to be very angry at Jean. Why are you so angry?

CRITIC: I hate her. She doesn't deserve to live. She's cursed. There's no point in trying to do anything with her. She is just cursed.

FACILITATOR: It sounds like you don't want her to be around.

CRITIC: I don't! I wish she would kill herself. I can't stand her.

FACILITATOR: Have you always felt this way or was there some point when all this started?

CRITIC: It's what happened with her father. She ruined my life when she let her father touch her. I hate her! I'll never forgive her for what she did.

Though the Inner Critic takes great pride in its rationality, once we separate from it we see just how irrational it is. In the case of the Killer Critic, we can often see the irrationality early in the game. Jean's, for instance, blames a six-year-old girl for the incest and will never forgive her. A Killer Critic hates us and can sometimes be recognized in expressions such as:

He's cursed.

She has poor genes.

He's a bad seed.

There's nothing there.

I want him dead.

She's a shell—there's just nothing inside her at all.

He's just hopeless, absolutely hopeless.

The more severe the abuse we suffer in our early life, the more likely it is that we have one of these Killer Critics. One central point is worth stressing: *It is absolutely possible to become aware of, to separate from, and to change a Killer Critic. It just takes a little more work.* We are dealing here with the Inner Abuser that is responsible for the continuing destruction of the Inner Child and the continuing ignition of the shame and abuse on an inner level. With a strong Critic, and particularly a Killer Critic, separating from shame and reclaiming the Inner Child are more difficult tasks.

Jean's Critic is particularly interesting because it blames her for everything. We can sense the deep shame, humiliation, and rage that this Critic experienced in regard to Jean's father. It feels that its life is truly ruined. It expresses itself in this way because there is no Aware Ego, no separation between Jean and the Critic. How can Jean lead any kind of creative life with this kind of attack going on inside of her? The answer is that she cannot. How can she feel adequate in any intimate relationship? The answer again is that she cannot.

The Aware Ego, when it begins to emerge, allows us to hear the voice of the Critic. We can listen to the attack. We can feel the desperate quality of the energy. At first we can merely identify the voice of the Critic, but with time, and as it grows stronger, we can begin to make changes. Ultimately, we can recognize the deep pain, humiliation, anxiety, and vulnerability that lie beneath the Critic and begin to become parent to it. It is strange to think of becoming parent to the Inner Critic. It is particularly strange to the Critic, itself. Nevertheless, this is the process we must follow. (For more information on learning to parent the Inner Critic, see chapter 17.)

PARTICULAR DANGERS OF A KILLER CRITIC

Killer Critics can cause serious depression, suicidal thoughts, and actual suicides. I (Hal) remember many years ago seeing a man with a Killer Critic. This was in the very beginning of the work with Voice Dialogue. I recommended to him that he do some journal writing on his own at home between himself and the Inner Critic. This is not something that I would do again under similar circumstances because we recognize now that the Killer Critic is too powerful to deal with in this way. The man returned for his next appointment a few days later and reported a dream he had the night of our session, the same night he did the writing. He dreamed of a black heart dripping black blood. This is what Killer Critics do to us. They cause severe depression.

Severe depression frequently accompanies a Killer Critic. A person being attacked by a Killer Critic is often unable to deal with people, work, and life in general. Relationships suffer profoundly because we cannot relate to others when this level of attack is going on within us much of the time. Therefore, support groups can be very important when a Killer Critic is operating, because people tend to feel isolated and these groups provide the human contact that is so necessary. When a Killer Critic is operating, appropriate therapeutic help and possibly antidepressant medication may well be indicated.

WHAT FACTORS GIVE RISE TO AND SUPPORT
THE KILLER CRITIC?

Many different kinds of life experiences give rise to a strong Critic in general and a Killer Critic in particular. Let us examine some of these factors now.

1. Abusive parents give rise to abusive Critics, as we said in the previous chapter. But there are some parents, one or both, who never wanted children or in some cases wanted to abort the child but could not, or simply were overwhelmed by the enormous demands of child rearing once the child was born. Their

inability to cope with these demands often causes much stress and anxiety. It is to be expected that these overwhelmed parents are frequently going to blame all their difficulties on the child and wish that the child was not there. They are very likely to tell this to the child. They make comments like:

If it weren't for you, everything would be OK.

I never wanted to have you in the first place.

Sometimes I wish that you never had been born.

I had a life before you came along.

Sometimes the parents move in the opposite psychological direction. For instance, an overwhelmed young mother might shift to acting like a totally devoted mother and repress the part of her that hates the child and really does not want to raise it. This underlying, unspoken attitude, together with the behavior and feelings that would accompany such child rearing, would naturally fatten up a Critic to killer proportions.

2. We frequently discover that serious physical or sexual abuse during childhood led to the development of a Killer Critic. This is illustrated in the conversation with Jean's Critic, which shows how a Killer Critic can develop in relationship to abusive sexuality in a family. One of the things that feeds the power of the Critic in these situations is the extended period of secrecy with its accompanying shame and guilt. *The longer the secrecy and silence of these situations, the stronger the Critic will become.*

3. The abuse that is committed through silence and withdrawal can also be devastating to a youngster, and the Killer Critic thrives in this kind of environment as well. Some people have an amazing capacity to punish with silence and withdrawal, and this creates fertile ground for Critic growth.

4. The overall lack of awareness in a person supports and maintains the power of the Critic. The Critic thrives on secrecy, on doing its work without our realizing it is there as a separate self. Any kind of therapy, self-help, or consciousness work that we do that enhances our awareness is going to help to neutralize the Critic at some level.

5. We often talk to the Killer Critics of people who spent their early lives in boarding schools or certain kinds of religious schools. These are very painful Voice Dialogue conversations because the persons experienced so much suffering in the growing-up process. In these settings certain people become the scapegoats of the teachers and students, and later in their lives the Killer Critics of these individuals take over this job of scapegoating with great authority.

DISOWNED INSTINCTUAL ENERGIES

The final factor that we are going to consider in the development of the Killer Critic is the disowning of our instinctual energies. Each of us is born with the capacity for certain kinds of feelings and certain kinds of behavior. These capacities are part of a genetic predisposition to act and behave in certain ways. We call them psychological instincts. Some instincts are totally physical in nature. Hunger, thirst, and sexuality would be examples of this. Other instincts tend to operate between the physical and the psychological. The capacity to behave aggressively in the world in order to get our needs met is an example of this. A more fully psychological instinct would be the capacity for parenting or higher wisdom.

Let us imagine that a youngster grows up in a family where aggression is not allowed to be present either in action or in thought. What happens to the child's anger? What happens to aggressive impulses? They are, after all, energy, and energy does not disappear. Blocked aggressive energy goes into the unconscious. It becomes a disowned energy system. At a certain point in the buildup of these negative energies we give them a different name. Instead of just calling them disowned instinctual energies, we now call them *daemonic* energies. We use this term to indicate the fact that these energies have shifted in a very special way. They have now become sour and destructive. Natural aggression becomes destructive aggression. Natural sexuality becomes destructive sexuality.

In our book *Embracing Our Selves,* we reported the dream of a spiritually oriented man in his midforties. He dreams that he is trying to wrestle a drunk penis into a cold shower. His penis stands for his sexuality, which in its natural state was not drunk and out of control. Several decades of renouncing his instinctual energies had distorted his natural sexuality. It grew out of proportion, becoming more and more powerful, and soon it was out of control as though drunk on alcohol. More and more effort was needed to keep his sexual energies under control. They had become daemonic and now presented a real danger to him in his life.

To the primary parental selves, these feelings seem to become more and more dangerous and much more energy must be spent in keeping them unconscious. However, the disowned and possibly daemonic energies want redemption. They want to rejoin the family. They come to us in our dreams. They are the bad men who are chasing us, the criminals who are trying to break into our house, the dangerous adolescents who are trying to rape us, the monsters who frighten us, and the wild animals who prowl the canvas of our dreamscape.

It is then that a very interesting thing begins to happen, and it happens at quite an early age. These powerful feelings and emotions that are blocked from reaching out into the world begin to shift to another track. They were initially on the aggression track, and if allowed to operate they would be part of our power and forcefulness in the world. Instead they spill over into another track, the Inner Critic track, and then the Inner Critic is infused with all of the power of our disowned aggression and emotional energy.

With all of this daemonic energy available, it is no wonder that the Critic can easily shift over into Killer Critic. Such a Critic sounds absolutely daemonic in the way it attacks us. "I hate her! I despise her! I detest her! I detest everything about her! She is so weak it's pitiful!" This daemonic rage, this daemonic condemnation is in large measure the disowned instinctual energy of our lives.

Therefore, an important part of the healing and weight reduction program that we must put the Killer Critic on requires us to get in touch with our instinctual energies and learn how to use our aggression and power in the world. Unintegrated power feeds the Critic like a banquet. Dealing with the Inner Critic forces us ultimately to claim this power back. The Critic does not give it up easily.

THE KILLER CRITIC AND THERAPY

A Killer Critic may well require special help. Many of the self-help programs are valuable here because they give people support and insight and a community in which to do their work. These might include any of the Twelve-Step programs such as A.A., A.C.A., O.A., Al-anon, and CODA. The spiritual base of these programs, plus the sense of community they provide for people, can provide a strong support to people who are trying to wrestle with these powerful Critics.

Sometimes psychotherapy may be needed as well, and we urge you to seek this kind of help when necessary. *It is important to do whatever you need to do to get out from under the domination of the Inner Critic.* To have someone as a guide who knows something about the terrain of the Critic may serve you well.

Chapter Ten

The Differences Between the Inner Critic in Women and in Men

The Inner Patriarch is a powerful archetypal ally of the Inner Critic in women. The synergy of these two voices makes the average woman's Inner Critic more powerful than the average man's. The voice of the Inner Patriarch is so familiar that, much like station KRAZY, it played constantly and was not even noticed until the feminists started their writings about thirty years ago. This Inner Patriarch is the inner representation of the outer, societal beliefs in the inferiority of women, and it echoes all the judgments against women that are prevalent in our culture. With its biblical beginnings, it has the ring of absolute knowledge and unquestioned authority.

In our many years of working with Inner Critics, we have noticed some major differences between the Inner Critics we meet in women and those we meet in men. This chapter is not meant to be a scientific study about these differences or a commentary on whether they are biologically or environmentally determined. It is, rather, a summary of the differences that we have noted consistently and cross-culturally.

THE POWER OF THE INNER CRITIC IN WOMEN AND IN MEN

The major difference between women and men is subtly, but startlingly, summed up in a scene from the movie *Tootsie*, which starred Dustin Hoffman. In this scene, Hoffman is impersonating a woman. He walks past his reflection in a mirror, looks at himself self-consciously, and carefully, but inconspicuously, adjusts his girdle so that he will look better. This simple movement tells it all! Earlier in the movie, we have seen Dustin Hoffman dressed as a man. He is relaxed about his appearance and does not give it a thought. He dresses and behaves as he pleases and never seems concerned about the impression that he will make on others. He is sure that he will be accepted for who he is and not for what he looks like. He is comfortable with himself. As a man, we never see him look at himself in a mirror except perhaps to shave. As a woman, all this changes. It is obvious to us that, as a man, he does not suffer from the attacks of an Inner Critic. As a woman, he does!

For us, this scene illustrates the most striking difference between the Inner Critics of men and women that we have observed. *Women's Inner Critics are almost always more powerful and more persistent than men's. Historically, this difference seems to be the product of thousands of years of patriarchal thinking.* This patriarchal view of the world sees women as somehow inferior to men. We will talk more about how this belief system intensifies the power of women's Inner Critics later in this chapter.

THE INNER CRITIC VS. THE JUDGE

In the growing-up process, we usually develop either a strong Inner Critic who judges us or a strong Inner Judge who judges the world. They are the oppposite sides of the same coin. Historically speaking, it is the women who have developed the Inner Critic as a primary self and the men who have developed the Judge. Although this is not true in certain parts of the world and it is changing as the role of women changes, we still see this as a major difference between women and men.

It is quite common for women to remember their fathers as judgmental rather than self-critical. Sometimes fathers are overtly judgmental, and sometimes their judgments come as silent signals—as special looks or as a withdrawal of attention. When you are a daughter of a judgmental father (or judgmental mother) you will probably develop a very strong Inner Critic.

When the parental judgments are quite subtle you might not even think of them as judgments that affect you. For instance, Dawn's father never said anything negative to her directly, but he was a very judgmental man who judged others in her presence. He would compliment Dawn for being different from them. For instance, he would judge others for being lazy and then compliment her for being hardworking. As Dawn grew older, she developed a powerful Inner Critic who watched her carefully to make sure that she would never be like the people her father judged!

DIFFERENCES IN CONTENT OF THE CRITIC'S COMMENTS

In contrast to a man's Inner Critic, a woman's Inner Critic seems to feel a pressing need to "improve" the woman's appearance or behavior in order to make her acceptable to others. It also tends to focus far more upon her physical appearance than a man's Inner Critic focuses upon his. Again, the scene from *Tootsie* is a beautiful picture of this.

It is unusual for a man's Inner Critic to be concerned about his weight. It is just not an issue, unless there is some health-related reason for him to worry about it. It is equally unusual for a woman's Inner Critic *not* to be concerned about her weight. Weight, for women, is almost always an issue! A similar division is apparent around aging. Women's Inner Critics, in past years, have worried themselves sick about the physical signs of aging, while men's Inner Critics have not necessarily seen this as a problem. The talking mirror is constantly pointing out the lines in the faces of women. This is quite unusual behavior in men.

The Critic's emphasis upon a woman's looks is so extreme that we have given many examples of it in this book. Media and advertising campaigns support an already powerful Inner

Critic by letting the woman know what is wrong with her or by encouraging her to compare herself to other more beautiful, self-assured, or younger women. This sells products, but it also intensifies the Inner Critic's emphasis upon a woman's looks.

ABOUT SEXUALITY

One of the most fascinating contrasts that we have noticed between the content of men's and women's Inner Critics has to do with what they say about sexuality. Men's Critics are usually worried about performance and adequacy, while women's Critics are usually worried about appearance and affection.

Thus, in the area of sexuality, the woman's Inner Critic is concerned with her appearance and her ability to earn love. If her man has been with another woman, her Inner Critic wants to know, "Is she more attractive?" or "Does he love her more than he loves you?" Her Inner Critic wants her to be loved the most.

In contrast, the man's Inner Critic is more anxious about his performance. If his woman has been with another man, his Inner Critic will want to know, "Is he better sexually than you are?" or "Does she like what he does better than what you do?" The Critic wants the man to perform well sexually, to satisfy his woman.

In recent years, as women have been told that they should be able to experience great sexual enjoyment, the Critic as Comparer has begun to criticize women about the quality and frequency of their orgasms. This, however, is not necessarily a focus on their sexual performance and its impact upon others. It is more a concern about achieving a goal, about feeling that they are the equals of the women who can enjoy themselves sexually. Here the goal is a good orgasm. The Inner Critic of a woman does not ordinarily question whether or not she has satisfied her partner adequately. This is not usually an issue for women, just as weight is not usually an issue for men.

THE REACTION TO CRITIC ATTACKS: WITHDRAWAL VS. NEEDINESS

We have noticed that men and women seem to react differently to Critic Attacks. The Inner Critic makes both men and women feel vulnerable. Men tend to deny this vulnerability and to deny that they care about what others think. They may feel it underneath, but they pull back from it. They then withdraw from contact with others. Women, in contrast, are more likely to reach out for reassurance and for contact with others to help lessen the feelings of isolation and misery that accompany a Critic Attack. In short, *in the face of a Critic Attack, men are likely to withdraw and women are likely to become needy.*

Let us see what this looks like in a typical interaction. Marv has had a bad day at work. As he drives home, his Inner Critic attacks him mercilessly, reviewing all the mistakes he made and letting him know that his boss probably thinks he is a hopeless idiot. Marv feels terrible and really worries about what the others at the office think of him, but he denies these feelings and pushes them deep down inside of him. Like many other men, Marv withdraws and becomes isolated when he can no longer bear the pain of the Critic Attack. When he finally arrives home, he is quiet and withdrawn. He says a brusque hello, takes the newspaper, and goes into the den to watch TV. He avoids Marian, his wife, and his children. They feel a bit abandoned and hurt, but they quickly group together and act as if nothing has happened, leaving Marv alone with his Critic and the TV. He feels isolated and miserable.

Marian has been well trained to take the blame for anything that goes wrong in her relationships. It is quite common for women to assume full responsibility for problems in relationship, and the Inner Critic supports this. Although she continues to go about her evening activities as usual, Marian feels vulnerable because Marv has withdrawn from her. She does not know it, but her Critic is already at work inside of her, questioning what it was that she did wrong to provoke Marv's grumpy withdrawal. Marian begins to feel uneasy and guilty. She is certain that she must have done something wrong, and her Inner Critic is busy reviewing the events of the last twenty-four hours in order to find out what that might be. Perhaps she was not interested enough this morning when Marv wanted to talk about the important meeting he was going to attend today; perhaps he was angry because last night she stayed up late to read and he might have wanted to have sexual relations, and so forth. The Inner Critic can come up with lots of creative reasons why others are angry with us!

If Marian feels guilty enough in the face of this Critic Attack, Marv will certainly flip to the other side of the coin and become judgmental of her. His Judge will be only too happy to agree with her Critic that his bad mood is all her fault! This will give him relief from his Critic Attack. He has already pushed down his own feelings of shame, he has flipped from Critic to Judge, and now he knows that his bad feelings are Marian's fault, not his.

In the face of her Critic Attack, Marian, like most women, is inclined to look around for affection and support rather than to withdraw from others. She becomes needy rather than isolated. First she will try to make contact with Marv, to get some reassurance that he still loves her. If this does not work, and it is likely that it will not, she may turn to her children or she may talk with friends. In talking to her friends, she may review the events of the evening and seek their reassurance that she did nothing wrong. She will try to get them to ally with her against the accusations of her Inner Critic. If this is successful, she will feel much better. She will have gotten the contact she needed, and she will have reassured her Inner Critic that she is not really a bad person. With the support of her friends, she might have flipped from Critic to Judge, just like Marv did, blaming him for everything "because he has always been such a moody, difficult man."

This is an ordinary occurrence; it is not the sign of a pathological relationship. We can see how both Marv and Marian were so badly hurt by the attacks of their Inner Critics that they were unable to reach out and to help one another. They could not use their relationship as a source of support and nourishment. If he had been aware of the activities of his Inner Critic, Marv might have been able to say, "I'm in the middle of a Critic Attack. It's nothing you've done. Something happened at the office and I just need you to love me and pay attention to me." If Marian's Critic had not been so quick to blame her for what was happening, she might have been able to reach out and comfort Marv.

This willingness of the Inner Critic to blame Marian for anything that goes wrong in relationship is one of the legacies of several thousand years of patriarchal thought. Let us now look further at the effect of the patriarchy on the Inner Critics of the women raised in our culture.

THE PATRIARCHY AND THE INNER CRITIC IN WOMEN

Women in our society have a distinct advantage when it comes to developing a truly enormous Inner Critic. Thousands of years of living under a patriarchal system have taught women that they are inferior to men and that no matter how hard they try they will always be basically inferior. The best that they can hope for is to become more like men—to pattern themselves on male role models and move away from their female instinctual behavior. In this effort to become something other than who they are, the Inner Critic plays a truly major role. After all, it is the Critic's responsibility to see what is wrong with the woman so that it can be corrected.

As the ad says, "You've come a long way, baby." Much has changed in women's roles and in the societal perceptions of women. But a five-thousand-year-old legacy does not disappear overnight. Even women who have lived independent lives as the equals of men often have within themselves, lurking deep in the shadows, an Inner Patriarch who echoes the sentiments of the outer patriarchs of the world. It is this Inner Patriarch, a most powerful archetype, who allies so strongly with the Inner Critic in most women.

EVER SINCE EVE

The view of woman as the inferior being, the first sinner, and as the one responsible for the fall of man and his expulsion from the Garden of Eden is clearly established in the first book of the Old Testament. Because of Eve's misbehavior, women are forever cursed by God: "Unto the woman he said, I will greatly multiply thy sorrow and thy conception; in sorrow thou shalt bring forth children: and thy desire shall be to thy husband, and he shall rule over thee" (Gen. 3:16, KJV).

It was the woman, Eve, who ate the apple from the tree of knowledge, and it was because of her that Adam and all men were cursed as well. "And unto Adam he said, *Because thou hast hearkened unto the voice of thy wife,* and hast eaten of the tree, of which I commanded thee saying, Thou shalt not eat of it: cursed is the ground for thy sake; in sorrow shalt thou eat of it all the days of thy life; thorns also and thistles shall it bring forth to thee; and thou shalt eat the herb of the field: in the sweat of thy face shalt thou eat bread, till thou return unto the ground . . ." (Gen. 3:17–19, KJV, italics ours). So this makes woman the source of all man's sorrows as well as those of her own.

No matter how you interpret this, no matter how religious you may be, if you are a woman raised anywhere in the Western world, this is a part of your heritage. This archetype is deep within your psyche. It is something shameful that your Inner Critic must help you to clear out. It was your fault!

You might also note two major aspects of the curse put upon woman. Both take away from her pride in herself and her ability to trust herself, thereby giving the Inner Critic even more cause for anxiety than it already has. First, God himself has stated that her husband must rule over her. It seems that he has better judgment than she has even though he too ate the fruit. Second, her very special gift, the ability to bring forth children, is cursed, and she is told that she must bring them forth in sorrow rather than in joy. This all helps to add serious amounts of weight to a woman's critic.

Since most of us are raised in religions that incorporate ancient biblical beliefs and traditions, we can assume that these traditions have a major impact upon our current beliefs and values whether or not we are consciously aware of them. As a Jewish woman, I (Sidra) was deeply shocked when my young daughter told me that the following prayer was said each morning by the boys in her Hebrew school. This prayer is from a current prayer book.

> Blessed art thou, O Lord our God, King of the
>   universe, who hast not made me a heathen.
> Blessed art thou, O Lord our God, King of the
>   universe, who hast not made me a bondman.
> *Blessed art thou, O Lord our God, King of the uni-*
>   *verse, who hast not made me a woman* [italics ours].

This is a pretty graphic picture of the low position in life accorded to women. Need we say more?

THE PATRIARCH WITHIN

What do we mean when we say the Inner Patriarch? We mean the voice in each of us, men and women alike, that views life in a patriarchal fashion. The Inner Patriarch basically values all things traditionally considered masculine and devalues things traditionally considered feminine. It thinks that men are better than women. Period!

The Inner Patriarch has clearly delineated sex roles, and these usually keep the woman in an inferior position. This does entitle her to protection, but in the eyes of the patriarch the woman is not seen as a fully developed human being who deserves the same rights as men or would be able to handle them responsibly if she were given them. Traditionally in our society, a woman was considered the property of her husband (or her father or her brother) and was not allowed to own property or in any way to act independently. It was only in this century that women were granted the right to vote. In America, we still cannot pass an equal rights amendment that would entitle women to little more than equal pay for equal work.

The Inner Patriarch is a powerful archetypal ally of the Inner Critic in women. The synergy of these two voices makes the average woman's Inner Critic more powerful than the average man's. The voice of the Inner Patriarch is so familiar that, much like station KRAZY, it played constantly and was not even noticed until the feminists started their writings about thirty years ago. This Inner Patriarch is the inner representation of the outer, societal beliefs in the inferiority of women, and it echoes all the judgments against women that are prevalent in our culture. With its biblical beginnings, it has the ring of absolute knowledge and unquestioned authority.

Many feminist writers focused on the outer patriarchs, the people and institutions in the culture that carried the patriarchal values and devalued women and all things womanly. These writers changed consciousness profoundly. Age-old "truths" were examined and found invalid. Women proved capable of reasoning, of successfully completing advanced degrees, of earning a living, of "making it" in a man's world. They entered fields that would have been closed to them a generation earlier. Feminists also brought attention to the fact that womanly activities such as childbearing and child rearing, caring for the home, and educating the young were considered inferior activities. They questioned the basic values of a society that valued competition (seen as patriarchal) as opposed to cooperation (seen as matriarchal).

The feminist scholars and writers brought forward a new and exciting body of knowledge for women. They challenged the system and changed the outer patriarchy in many areas. But what they did not notice was that there was an enemy within. *Within most women is an Inner Patriarch who believes that she is* indeed inferior and that she needs constant surveillance to keep her behavior appropriate! It feels a deep-seated disdain for her femaleness and can literally make her ashamed to be a woman. This Patriarch allies itself with the woman's Inner Critic for a great double whammy.

What about women who have freed themselves of the restrictions of the outer patriarchy? Some women have taken the step of fully incorporating male values and succeeding in a man's world. In some of them, the Inner Patriarch takes an interesting form: these women feel good about themselves but superior to the woman who has remained more traditionally feminine. They belittle the housewife and mother, seeing her choice in life as an inferior one. Thus they assume the role of the Patriarch and make patriarchal judgments without realizing that they have actually become the hated enemy!

It is easier to fight an enemy outside than an enemy within. It is important for women to know that an Inner Patriarch exists within them, that patriarchy is not just an enemy to be battled on the outside. For many women, this is a revelation. They have been so busy with the outer battles, which have been monumentally important, that they have not necessarily looked within. As Pogo said, "We have met the enemy and he is us."

What does this "enemy" look like? The Inner Patriarch knows that you will never make it in this world just because you are a woman. The Critic's job, then, is even more difficult, and its underlying anxiety is increased. Not only do you have many shortcomings and basic flaws as a human being, but you are also a woman! Your Critic may feel that the only way in which you can succeed in this world is if it makes you less of a woman, and so it will be alert to any natural "feminine" impulses and will do its best to rid you of them. At best, your Critic has a huge job.

WHAT DOES THE INNER PATRIARCH SAY TO WOMEN?

We were introduced to the Inner Patriarch in Holland when I (Sidra) started to run a women's group as part of a larger workshop. Something was wrong, very wrong. The women who had been animated and excited just moments before were quiet and even a bit sullen. I suddenly felt as though I were sitting in a room of judgmental men. At that moment I asked if the women were unhappy about being with women only. The answer was definitely yes. The women in the group felt that nothing important could come from a group that contained only women and that it was presumptuous for a woman (Sidra) to think that she or any woman, for that matter, had anything important to say. The Inner Patriarchs of the group were then addressed and had a chance to air their views of women.

Like the Dutch women, it is important for others as well to stop for a moment and listen to what their Inner Patriarchs have to say. Many of the following statements are deeply embedded in our culture and may seem like ordinary everyday truths to you. Let us listen to some of the comments of the Inner Patriarchs that we have heard over the years as taken from Voice Dialogue transcripts. Many of the women whose Patriarchs are quoted below hold professional positions in which they wield great authority and power. The Inner Patriarch could care less.

Women should not be in any position of power because it violates the natural order of things.

She's a woman and she will never amount to much. It's ridiculous for her to even hope for anything. Basically, she's better off not trying.

It's too bad she was born a woman. If only she were a man, she could make better use of her brains (or physical prowess, sports ability, common sense, natural aggressiveness, etc.).

If she does develop her natural power and she gets anywhere professionally, she will still be a woman. She can't escape that.

The planet is falling apart because women are deserting their natural roles.

The best thing for a woman to do is find herself a good husband and settle down.

I hate to have to work with women. I much prefer men.

Women are bitchy and nagging underneath. They complain too much.

Women should stop pretending to be men. They should stay home and get married and stop wanting more.

Women's hormonal imbalances make them unfit for any serious responsibilities.

Frankly, I think a woman's job is to get a rich husband so that she'll be able to take care of her parents when they get older.

Women are too emotional and are always overreacting.

Women are illogical.

Women have no mathematical ability.

Women lack focus.

Women have no real sense of values; they're frivolous.

I can't stand women's talk. It has no substance.

Women are basically weaker than men.

Just give them some good sex and they'll shut up.

Women are irresponsible. When it comes to important things they are not to be trusted.

You can never really understand a woman.

I'm a thinker. Women can't think clearly. They just pretend that they can.

Women are too needy.

I don't want children, that's for women!

Women are gullible and have very poor judgment.

Basically, there's only one thing they're really good for and that's sex.

Once a woman is no longer attractive and good for sex, she is basically worthless.

THE IMPORTANCE OF RECOGNIZING THE INNER PATRIARCH

It is amazing to realize that a voice in a woman could make these kinds of statements without the woman having any idea that this process is happening. We have seen women battered over and over again by the outer patriarchs in their lives, and they are either victims to it or they become rebellious daughters to it. The war goes on, year after year and decade after decade, until finally the realization comes that the problem is within as well as without. It is also important to recognize that this patriarchal voice can manifest in a male authority figure or a female authority figure and that a woman can be the victim of either one.

No amount of battling with the patriarchs outside can compensate for the damage done by your own Inner Patriarch. It is time to turn the attention within and to deal with your own Patriarch. After all, if your Patriarch did not basically agree with the criticisms of the world outside, they would have little effect upon you. If your Critic were not afraid that you are, indeed, inferior because you are a woman, then the judgments of others would have less impact.

If you, as a woman, can begin to hear the voice of the Patriarch within, you will find that his comments are responsible for a deep-seated feeling of shame that seems to have no particular focus. It is the shame of being a woman in this culture. As you separate from your Inner Patriarch, you will begin to see him change. At some point, the Inner Patriarch may well assume a more positive role in your life, using his masculine power to support you from within. You will hear his deep-seated concern for your well-being and for the problems that you face in what remains an essentially patriarchal society that he knows only too well.

THE INNER MATRIARCH AND THE INNER CRITIC

Many men have mentioned that it is not only women who have problems with an archetypal ally of the Inner Critic. They point out that men often have a judgmental Inner Matriarch who works with their Critic and who despises them just because they are men. We have found that this is more likely among younger men and that it usually is not as destructive as the patriarchal aspects of the Critic are to women. The matriarchal voices have been somewhat silent (or at least hidden) for many centuries, and they are far less virulent in our dominant culture. However, in some areas, the matriarchal voices are being heard again and the presence of the Inner Matriarch is becoming more prevalent than it used to be. Men who have been raised in a matriarchal setting, with little or no masculine input, often have an Inner Matriarch who does not like them just because they are men and who judges them disdainfully. Some of the Inner Matriarch's comments we have heard are as follows:

Men are impossible.

Oh, you know men. They're are all such babies underneath!

Men are responsible for the mess the world is in today.

Men are too aggressive.

You can't really talk to a man.

All they want is sex.

If it wasn't for needing children I would be very happy without men in the world. Women are so much more caring.

I don't really like men. I like women better.

Men are necessary as studs, nothing more.

The trouble with men is they are too rational or they are never in touch with their feelings or they cannot be trusted.

A truly virulent Inner Matriarch can be as destructive as an Inner Patriarch and must be separated from. It is important to take this deep-seated poison out of the system when dealing with the Inner Critic, because until you do so, the Inner Patriarch and the Inner Matriarch will continue to provide fuel and power for the Inner Critic and make your job of separation that much harder.

DISEMPOWERING THE INNER PATRIARCH AND THE INNER MATRIARCH

Separating from the Inner Patriarch and the Inner Matriarch, voices that usually operate with the support of the culture in which we live, is extremely liberating. *To separate means to hear what these voices say and to realize that they represent selves that have a particular point of view but do not necessarily bear an ultimate truth.* It is fairly simple to see that your Critic is criticizing you unrealistically if you hear your neighbor's Inner Critic criticizing her for the opposite "sin," like being too ordinary or too special or being too aggressive or too passive. But when everyone's Inner Patriarch more or less agrees with everyone else's, you do not have external points of reference to check against. This is why we have included this chapter and its exercises. This chapter gives you that external point of reference to check against.

Disempowering these archetypal voices can lessen the size and power of the Critic and make it more manageable. There's an age-old tradition in dealing with an overwhelming enemy: it is divide and conquer. That is just what we are doing when we separate from the Inner Patriarch and Matriarch. Then the Aware Ego can deal with each of these energies separately from those of the Inner Critic instead of having to battle them all at once.

◆ WHAT DOES YOUR INNER PATRIARCH SAY?

The realization of how your Inner Patriarch (or Matriarch) contributes to your Inner Critic and the knowledge of its roots in your culture and your personal life gives you important information and objectivity in dealing with its comments.

1. What does *your* Inner Patriarch say?

As you finish this chapter, see if you can tune into the voice of your Inner Patriarch. Write down the negative comments that your Inner Patriarch makes about women. Begin them with "women are . . ." You may repeat statements that you have read here if they feel familiar to you. Leave a space next to each of these comments so that you can make an additional notation.

2. What does your Inner Matriarch say?

Tune into the voice of your Inner Matriarch. Write down the negative observations that your Inner Matriarch makes about men. Begin them with "Men are . . ." Leave a space next to each of these comments so that you can make an additional notation.

3. Now, next to each comment, write down its source. For instance, was it something your father or mother used to say? Did you hear this from a teacher? advisor? employer? brother? sister? If you cannot specify a specific source, just write "cultural." This will give you some indication of where these judgments originated in your life.

4. Now that you have begun to hear the voice of your Inner Patriarch, you are in a position to separate from it. Look at the comments of your Inner Patriarch. Remember that even if a comment represents an idea that everyone in your community agrees is valid, "it ain't necessarily so." It might be helpful to have some contact with someone who already knows about the Inner Patriarch to help you as you separate from yours. Reading books by some of the feminist writers (or by men who are trying to raise the consciousness of men) will help you to get some separation from the ideas held as sacred by your archetypal Inner Patriarch (or Matriarch).

THREE

The Inner Critic and Relationship

Chapter Eleven

The Critic as a Relational Creature

"What will people think?" This is one of the Critic's favorite questions. The Inner Critic, as you may have noticed, is constantly looking at others to figure out who you should be. There is no deep introversion here, no looking within to find out what is important to you as an individual human being. The Critic's bottom-line concern is the impression that you will make upon others.

The Inner Critic is a relational creature, a truly people-oriented self. It develops out of our relationships with others. As we demonstrated in chapter 1, the Inner Critic learns a great deal from our parents, and it is ever alert to our interpersonal interactions. It seems to observe us through the eyes of the world around us and is particularly concerned about the impact that our actions have on others.

"WHAT WILL PEOPLE THINK?"

"What will people think?" is one of the Critic's favorite questions. The Inner Critic, as you may have noticed, is constantly looking out at others to figure out who you should be. There is no deep introversion here, no looking within to find out what is important to you as an individual human being. The Critic's bottom-line concern is the impression that you will make upon others.

Underneath it all, the Critic is usually afraid of being unloved, abandoned, and helpless. It wants to ensure that others will approve of you, love you, and be there for you when you need them. Or perhaps the Critic is not as interested in affection as it is in power and the admiration of others. It hopes that people will be attracted to you because you are powerful, interesting, or brilliant and you will never have to worry about being alone and helpless.

"What will people think?" is often what your parents asked, either aloud or by implication. They wanted you to be appropriate and to think of the consequences of your actions. This was for their sakes as well as for your own. After all, your behavior directly reflected your parents' performance. It showed whether or not they did a good job raising you. If you are a good person or a success, you are a credit to them. If you are a bad person or a failure, they will be blamed. So you carry with you not only your own requirements for acceptance, but your parents' feelings too. This is quite a task for your Inner Critic.

The concern with what others will think includes not only people but God as well. For those of us with a more spiritual background, it is extremely important to behave as God wishes us to. The Inner Critic takes on the task of making sure that we lead the right kind of life so that our relationship with God is a good one. It must then point out to us all the ways in which we have been falling short of this goal.

We have noticed three major reasons for wanting to lead a spiritually correct life and maintain a proper relationship to God. First of all, many of us believe it is simply the right way to be. The rules are clear and it is up to us to follow them. If this is our approach, then the Critic supports us by bringing to our attention all the ways in which we are falling short of living the proper kind of life. It wants to help us remain on the proper path. Second, many of us feel a deep love for God and need to remain in touch with divinity at all times. If we do not, then we feel an irreplaceable loss and a lack of meaning in life. The Inner Critic is usually not active when this kind of motivation is operating. However, if the Critic is active, it will attack us for not following the kind of program that keeps us in touch with divinity (such as regular prayer or meditation) and will tell us that we know better than to neglect our spiritual practices. Third, there is the issue of the hereafter. Many Inner Critics take on the awesome responsibility of keeping us in a good relationship with God so that when the final judgment comes we will not be found wanting. It is surprising how often we find Inner Critics who are very concerned with our making it to heaven, even in people who rejected their traditional religious upbringing and practices early in their lives.

The following surprising portion of a Voice Dialogue conversation with Milly's Inner Critic powerfully conveys its concern with what other people will think and what God will think.

FACILITATOR: We've been talking to you for a while now, and it's obvious that it is very important for you that Milly is a good person. It seems to really upset you when she isn't.

CRITIC: Yes. That's the way it should be. I don't even see what there is to talk about. I don't like it at all when she's not good or even when she has mean thoughts. Her parents were good people, they didn't have mean thoughts, and they tried to raise her to be a good girl. They did everything that they could and they set a very good example. They were not hypocrites!

FACILITATOR: I was wondering if there is anything else that you are particularly worried about. (The Critic had already told the facilitator that Milly's family was very religious, and the facilitator wondered whether the Critic was worried about what would happen to Milly after death.)

CRITIC: I don't want anybody to say anything bad about her parents. I've always tried hard to make them proud of her so that they'll feel good about themselves. I told you, they tried real hard. They deserve to feel proud of themselves.

FACILITATOR: I know. But I have a feeling that there's something else, something underneath. What is it?

CRITIC (begins to cry): I want Milly to get to heaven, that's for sure, but what I'm really afraid of is that if Milly is bad, her parents won't get into heaven. And that wouldn't be fair. They're such good people and they deserve it, and I wouldn't want them hurt because of something that she has done. Wouldn't that be awful?

THE INNER CRITIC HAS DEVELOPED IN RELATIONSHIP

Since it has its beginnings in relationship, the Inner Critic is basically an other-directed social creature. It developed in relationship, and it continues to operate prominently in all our relationships, even when we are not aware of it. Its deep interpersonal roots were originally fed by the judgments of the important people in our lives. We either developed Critics that echoed the judgments of our primary caretakers, or we rebelled and developed Critics that took the opposite point of view, making us very different from these primary caretakers.

Let us see how this works. Andy comes from a tightly knit family that is loyal, loving, and responsible. They seem to live a good life, and they have many friends. People respect them, and this is very important to them. Andy learns from his parents that it is important to be a good, responsible, cooperative, dependable person. His parents are harsh in their judgments of any selfish or irresponsible behavior. They frequently talk about old Uncle Silas who was very different from their side of the family. Silas was more of a loner and always put his own needs first. As Silas carried their disowned selves, Andy's parents judge him for having lived life the wrong way. They are quick to point out that he died alone and unloved because he was such a selfish, inconsiderate person. Nobody, but nobody, would want to be like that!

In order to fit in, to win their admiration and their love, Andy develops a set of primary selves that match the primary selves of his family. He too becomes a loving, loyal, and responsible person. His Critic sees to it that anything that might seem disloyal, irresponsible, or selfish is deleted from his thoughts and his feelings—and most certainly from his actions.

His Inner Critic works from the inside, criticizing any thoughts or feelings that might displease his family, so that anything that would be inappropriate in this family system is disowned even before it can come to the surface. The Inner Critic makes Andy feel terrible whenever he shows any indication of being like Uncle Silas, even just a little bit. We might think of his Critic as a kind of psychological house cleaner who tidies up and gets rid of any unsightly emotions or inclinations.

Andy's Inner Critic works with the primary selves of Responsible Father and Cooperative Son, and Andy is happily accepted into his family as a good person. He is loved and he is not alone. But he has paid his price; he has disowned any parts of himself that do not fit this happy picture. His Critic, having learned his lesson well, will see to it that Andy is a Responsible, Dependable Father and a Cooperative Son in his future relationships as well, especially in relation to his wife and children.

In contrast to Andy, Anna develops a set of primary selves that are the opposite of those of her family of origin. Her parents are incompetent and have no control over their lives. Nobody admires them. They drink a good deal, fight with one another, have an untidy household, and have no real friends. Anna sees that this does not work very well and looks around to find other, better examples to follow. She judges her parents as being wrong in the way they approach life and develops a set of primary selves that are the opposite of theirs. *Her primary selves, instead of helping her in her relationship to her family, help her in relationship to the world.* They help her to fit into the bigger world, the one in which her parents do not function effectively. Somehow, Anna seems to have realized that she will never be able to get her needs for nurturance and safety met in her household, no matter what she might do.

Anna is fortunate that she reacts to her dysfunctional family in this way. Rather than become like her family, she learns to avoid their errors. Perhaps she has a grandparent, an aunt, a teacher, a friend, or a friend's family to provide her with an alternative model of behavior. Perhaps she learns from watching others on television. Basically, she does not try to fit into the family system. Instead, she withdraws from it. Psychologists have tried to explain why some people react like Anna by becoming strong in the face of adversity and some do not. We are not aware of any definitive answers to this question at this time.

Anna becomes a managing type of woman—a leader and an organizer. She likes being in charge of everything and at the center of the action. She is always busy. Her primary selves are competent and controlling. Anna's Inner Critic is terrified that she will collapse into incompetence if she ever slows down. Its greatest fear is that she will become like her parents. So it always keeps her in the roles of manager and of the initiator in relationship. It criticizes her when she is emotional (because it remembers her parents' fights), and it does not allow her to feel needy so that she will not be disappointed in case nobody is there to take care of her. Her Critic makes her ashamed of any signs of weakness, of anything less than a Wonder Woman approach to life.

We can expect the Inner Critic to continue to control Anna in this way and to have a significant effect upon her relationships. Her Critic will tell her that she should not be weak or passive and that she must stay in control of all her relationships. She should not relax and take from others, because this could prove dangerous. The overall effect is that Anna must, in all of her relationships, assume the active role and remain the initiator. She will, of course, find herself surrounded by needy, ineffectual people who will need her to dominate them and take care of them.

In both Andy's and Anna's stories, we can see how the Inner Critic developed in relationship to their families and how these Critics will continue to guide their relationships in the future. Andy's Inner Critic keeps him responsible, dependable, and unselfish, and Anna's keeps her strong, busy, and in control. Neither Inner Critic gives them an opportunity to express their inner needs or feelings in a direct manner. Each Inner Critic keeps the focus upon behaving appropriately, that is, in line with the requirements of the primary selves. Neither Anna nor Andy has any way of contacting the Inner Child and taking care of it consciously because its emotions, needs, and general vulnerability are considered taboo by the Critic. The Inner Child is seen as a hindrance to relationship or to functioning in general.

As a final example, let us consider Randy. His mother and father are perfectionistic, so much so that it is almost impossible to match their expectations. So Randy does not. He does not even like the way they are, so why should he try to be like them? As a matter of fact, he would be much better off going in the opposite direction. And so he does. Instead of becoming perfectionistic, Randy rebels against his parents' requirements. He becomes quite relaxed, even sloppy, in his approach to life. "Be cool," he often says as he tries to get people to relax. His primary selves judge people who are too uptight; they feel that perfectionism is foolish. They think that life is to be enjoyed and that spending time on making life perfect is wasteful.

Randy's primary selves, then, are the disowned selves of the family. *Instead of his Inner Critic trying to make him fit into his family (like Andy's) and judging him if he deviates from his family's requirements, his primary selves judge his parents for their foolish perfectionism.* Randy's Inner Critic, however, would judge him if he tried to be perfect. It would say something like, "You're acting just like your mother. How disgusting!" Under conditions of real stress, such as the loss of a job, the Critic is quite capable of reversing roles and criticizing him for being too sloppy, even though this is not its primary orientation.

Like Anna, Randy's primary selves are the disowned selves of his family. Both Randy and Anna judge their parents for what they are like. But their primary selves have developed to serve two different functions. Anna's primary selves protect her vulnerability by specifically trying to enable Anna to fit into society. In contrast, Randy's primary selves are protecting his Vulnerable

Child from the pain of trying to accomplish something impossible. There is no way that Randy can be as perfect as his parents wish him to be! His primary selves make sure that he does not even try, and thus there is no way that he can fail.

THE INNER CRITIC AS EVALUATOR OF OUR READINESS FOR RELATIONSHIP

By now, you have seen how much vested interest the Inner Critic has in your relationships. Next, we would like to introduce you to another role that the Inner Critic can play in relationship, a role that historically is rather a new one. Years ago, people entered primary relationships simply because it was time to do so. There was no concern about anyone's readiness for relationship. It was assumed that if you were interested, you were ready. Since divorce has become so common and it has become apparent over the last twenty-five years that not everyone is ready, many people wonder whether or not they are truly ready for relationship. And guess who is likely to answer the question "Am I ready for a lasting relationship?" You're right, it is the Inner Critic.

Underneath the Inner Critic feels vulnerable. It is panicked that you will mess up, that you will prove unacceptable when someone really moves in close to you, that your relationship will not last, and that you will ultimately be abandoned. So it sets out to examine all systems before it will allow you to take the chance of commitment. When an Inner Critic is the evaluator of readiness, you can imagine what happens. It is quite unlikely that you will ever pass its test!

And so your Inner Critic tells you that you are just not ready. First, your physical appearance is not yet up to par. You must lose weight, exercise more and get rid of your flab, lose that cellulite, dye your hair, fix your nose, and possibly get a face-lift. You do not have your work act together. Before you think of a committed relationship, get yourself a better job so that you will be able to afford a family. Get another degree. You are not sexy enough. You are still too boring. You are not emotionally ready. You must get your psyche in order so that you will not allow yourself to get into another codependent situation. You have not learned how to be intimate. You do not know how to be separate. You cannot set appropriate boundaries. You are not responsible enough. You are too responsible. And on and on it goes.

Some of its comments may have objective value, of course, but it is the feeling behind them that counts. The message that it puts across is that you, as a human being, are just not enough. You must be improved upon before you are fit for relationship with another human being. If, however, you wait for the Inner Critic to let you know that you are ready, you are in big trouble. We sincerely doubt that it will ever give you the go-ahead signal.

This readiness for relationship includes the readiness for parenthood. Having a baby is taking an irrevocable step into relationship. It involves a lifetime of responsibility and, needless to say, the Inner Critic panics because it fears failure in this all-important venture. A new generation of Inner Critics have grown fat with all the new knowledge about the damage that parents do when they parent poorly. The Inner Critic of many psychologically sophisticated individuals is quick to say:

You're not ready to have a child.

You have a lot to clear up in yourself before you could possibly think of taking on responsibility for someone else.

You have a whole lifetime of inner work to do before you will be in a position to parent effectively.

You certainly don't plan to put your children through the same discomfort that you have had to suffer. You don't want to be the kind of parent that your parents were.

So you can see that the Inner Critic is a part of you that is almost always thinking in terms of relationship. Now, let us move forward and explore its role more deeply. First, we will look at how the Inner Critic is affected by the judgments of others. Then we will show you how its actions directly sabotage your relationships. Last, we will see how a hyperactive Inner Critic makes intimacy impossible.

◆ HOW DOES YOUR INNER CRITIC WANT YOU TO RELATE TO OTHERS?

The following exercises will help you to see how your Inner Critic and your primary selves want you to relate to others. Remember, these selves originally evolved to protect you in your family of origin. With this new information and objectivity, your Aware Ego can look at their current effect on your life and relationships and can begin to modify their power if they are no longer serving you properly. In this way, your Aware Ego can take over the function of protection that was formerly served by these primary selves.

How does the Critic behave in relation to your primary selves? If your primary selves match those of your parents, your Critic will criticize you for any deviation from these selves. In order to protect you in your relationships, it will try to keep you relating to your parents and to the other people in your life just the way your parents do. If, however, your primary selves are the opposite of your parents, your Inner Critic will generally criticize you if your behavior in any way resembles theirs. Then it will try to protect you in relationship by ensuring that your actions are the opposite of theirs. Your Inner Critic does not want you to take any chances in life or in relationships, so it basically supports your old patterns of behavior even as it criticizes you for having them.

1. What will people think? Try to tune into the voice of your Inner Critic to hear its fears about what people will think. See if you can come up with your Critic's favorite "people will think" statements. Perhaps these statements sound like ones that your parents used to make. Some common statements are:

People will think you don't know anything.

People will think you are selfish.

People will think you're bossy.

People will think you're not nice.

People will think you have no manners.

2. Are you basically a spiritual or religious person? If so, does your Inner Critic worry about your relationship to God? What are its major concerns?

3. Are your primary selves like your parents? Think of Andy's story. Which of your primary selves are like either of your parents?

4. Which of your primary selves are the opposite of your parents? For instance, if your parents were noisy, are you quiet?

5. What does your Critic say about your readiness for relationship? Or, if you are in a relationship already, where does it see your inadequacies?

6. Look at your primary selves and reevaluate their roles. Consider your primary selves as you defined them in this exercise and the one in chapter 1. Are there ways in which your primary selves no longer work for you? Think about the last time one of your primary selves automatically took over in your relationship and it caused a problem. Then think of a possible alternate behavior that might have served you better. For instance, you may be very independent and never ask for help. Whenever you feel vulnerable, you get tough and self-sufficient. Last week, you needed assistance in moving some heavy boxes while you were cleaning out the garage, but because of your independence you refused to call your husband to ask him to help. Your Inner Critic said that if you called him, he would think you were a pest. So you lifted boxes that were too heavy and you hurt your back. You felt abandoned by him and you judged him angrily for never helping you when you really needed him. As you think of an example like this, you are using your Aware Ego to look at the roles played by your primary self and your Inner Critic. This makes you aware of your own behavior and creates the possibility of real choice in the future. Maybe next time

you feel the surge of self-righteous independence, you will stop for a moment and ask yourself if, perhaps, you need some help. Then you have the choice to ask for the help that you truly need in this situation.

Chapter Twelve

Growing Up in the Family
Disowned Selves, Judgment, and the Development of the Inner Critic

Whatever we disown in ourselves will be exactly the personality traits that come back to us in our relationships. Whatever we disown in ourselves, we will find in other people, and we will feel either a very strong judgment or a very strong attraction toward them. Since at some level we are all reflections of each others' disowned selves, it is inevitable that we will be judged by many of the people in our lives.

We have seen many examples of how the Inner Critic depends upon the judgments of other people for its proper development. We have also defined the Inner Critic as that part of ourselves that criticizes or judges us. On the other hand, the Judgmental Self is that part of us that criticizes other people or the part of other people that criticizes us. The reality of life is that we *are* judged frequently by others, and most of us, on some level, tend to be fairly judgmental of other people as well. In fact, the extent to which many of our relationships are dominated by judgment and self-criticism is truly remarkable!

In our chapter on Critic Attacks we examined some of the kinds of outer judgments that stimulate our Inner Critics. In this chapter we want to explore more deeply the role of judgment in our personal relationships. Specifically, we want to explore what happens to the child in the family interactional system. How and why do the judgments of parents develop, and how do they then feed into the child? In chapter 1 we presented a summary of certain basic principles that we are now going to review because they are important for understanding the patterns of family interactions.

DISOWNED SELVES AND PRIMARY SELVES

You will remember that in the growing-up process it is quite natural to identify with certain selves that, over time, begin to define our personality. These selves are basically protective. From an early age, they step in to regulate our behavior. They are protective because we are so vulnerable and so easily hurt. They do their best to keep us safe. These are the primary selves that are basically responsible for taking care of us.

Let us use the example of a little girl growing up in a chaotic and emotionally volatile family where it is essential for her to please people. Like many of us in similar situations, she develops a Pleaser as a primary self. This Pleaser is a very natural and powerful self that serves her in many ways. She believes that if she is nice to people, then they will be nice to her. Being nice to people keeps them happy and the waters stay smooth. Even though it may not always work, it works enough of the time to establish it as a primary pattern.

At the same time she may learn to be very responsible and to take care of her parents, siblings, and/or friends. Being very nice and taking care of people becomes a way of life for her that determines her behavior in every relationship that she has. In this process, she must naturally disown her "not nice" and "irresponsible" selves. This kind of pleasing and responsible behavior gets many of us through childhood safely and sometimes pleasantly and then becomes the basis for our adult personalities.

Because of the fact that major parts of ourselves must be disowned for the Pleaser to develop, some writers and teachers today refer to it as a "false self." The same kind of judgment is directed toward other kinds of selves that may have helped us in the growing-up process. An example of this would be the part of us that is nurturing and that always takes on responsibility for other people's actions.

We prefer not to call these selves false. This kind of judgment just feeds the Inner Critic. These selves are primary selves, parts of us that have done the best job that they could possibly do in raising and caring for us. They are quite ready to relinquish their hold over us when we have developed our awareness and our ability to handle the world in a different way. *Every primary self is waiting for the Aware Ego to be born so that it can go into semiretirement. Each is doing what must be done, protecting us in the world as best it can, until we learn how to do it for ourselves.* Once we no longer have to please people and be responsible for them, once we can handle the consequences of a new kind of behavior, then the older primary self can relax and take a well-earned vacation.

In this sense, our primary selves are like parents who have grown old and yet continue to give us the same kind of advice and to control our behavior in the same way as when we were quite young. As with our outer parents, so with our inner parents. When they finally feel that they can trust us and that we truly will be responsible for ourselves, and behave appropriately, then they are able to let go and allow us to lead our lives independently. When we talk to these primary selves in Voice Dialogue conversations, they usually feel that their way of operating in the world is the safest for the person, and their feelings are hurt when they are referred to as false or not real. This kind of language tends, in fact, to make them much more stubborn, more fixed in their ways, and less likely to relinquish control.

As we have seen, for every primary self that develops, there will be another part of us that is equal and opposite in intensity and that will not have a chance to express itself in our lives in a regular way. Although these disowned selves live quite unconsciously, they often break out at unexpected moments, much to the chagrin of the primary-self system.

So, in the example given above, if we develop a strong Pleaser in our style of dealing with the world, underneath there will be very selfish tendencies that rarely get a chance to emerge. If we identify with very strong and aggressive and powerful selves, then we will disown our vulnerability. If we grow up identified with a loving and caring way of being in the world, our disowned selves will be more aggressive, not nice, and possibly nasty. If we grow up being identified with our introversion, then our extraversion will be disowned. Many such opposites are possible.

It is impossible to escape the developing disowned selves. It is a totally natural and inevitable process. However, these disowned selves do bring about a set of consequences that we need to understand. Again we repeat what we said in chapter 1, because this idea is so basic to the understanding of human interactions. *Our primary selves are who we think we are!* If we grow up with primary selves that are strong and powerful, we think that we are strong and powerful. If we grow up being identified with sensitivity and feeling, we think that is who we are. We never realize that this particular way of being in the world is the expression of only one self or, more likely, one set of selves. When we use the word *I,* we are in fact referring to the primary selves, but we do not know this.

Now we come to the point that is essential in understanding the way our selves, and the Critic in particular, operate in relationships. *Whatever we disown in ourselves will be exactly the personality traits that come back to us in our relationships.* Whatever we disown in ourselves, we will find in other people, and we will feel either a very strong judgment or a very strong attraction toward them. Since in some way we are all reflections of each others' disowned selves, it is inevitable that we will be judged at some level by many of the people in our lives. As we said in our book *Embracing Our Selves,* every disowned self becomes one of God's little heat-seeking missiles making its way back toward us!

In the outer world, we hate and judge whatever it is that we disown, and we have no idea that this is happening. The opposite is also true. Our attractions and fascinations with things and people also tend to be expressions of our disowned selves. The emphasis here is, of course, on the judgments rather than the attractions because we are dealing with the development of the Critic.

When we make judgments based on our disowned selves, we feel righteously correct. Out of this feeling of righteousness, we can justify almost any way of acting or feeling toward the other person. Noticing whether or not we feel righteous helps differentiate between judging and discerning. When we judge, we are righteous. When we are discerning, we are objective.

Let us consider an example of this kind of judgment. Imagine that Jane is at a party with her husband. She is thirty-five years of age with three children and very much lives out a mother role in which she is responsible for children, husband, and friends. At the party is a woman about her own age who has had a considerable amount to drink and who is flirting outrageously with a number of men. To complete the picture, she is dressed in a sexy outfit with a very low neckline. Jane says to her husband, "That is the most disgusting sight I have ever seen!" This is a clear judgment. In her own life she has disowned her sensual energy. Flirting is not allowed because her Critic is still echoing her parents' voices, loud and clear, though she is not aware of this. From the time Jane was a little girl she was admonished for being sensual, and this admonishment continues on an inner as well as outer level. Jane must be proper. When she meets someone who is open and flirtatious and not proper, Jane's primary selves come into operation. They judge the behavior of the other person. The stronger the disowned selves, the stronger the judgment.

Yvonne is at the same party with her husband. She sees the same woman but she is not at all threatened, upset, or fascinated by her. She senses the woman is behaving inappropriately and has no particular desire to make contact with her, but she does not have a strong emotional reaction to this woman.

Yvonne is in touch with her sensuality. She is in touch with the part of her that knows how to be outrageous and that enjoys flirting, and so this is not an issue for her. She is able to make discernments about the person and situation because no disowned selves are operating.

Our judgments always have behind them a quality of righteousness. They convey an emotional impact, even when they are not spoken, and the person to whom they are directed always feels put down, no matter how subtle the judgment may be. Discernments are not righteous. They are much more impersonal and objective. There is no need to put the other person down in any way. This principle of judgment and the disowned selves is of the utmost importance in human relationship in general and in family settings in particular. Let us turn to some examples to see how these disowned selves affect the growing-up process.

THE GIVING MOTHER

Mary is best described as a giving mother. She is always available to her children and husband and friends. She developed this way of being in the world because it allowed her to survive a very painful childhood in which her own parents were not available to her. When she was a young child, her parents were gone a great deal of the time. She was left with baby-sitters constantly, and she remembers being terrified by the constant turnover of sitters and the feeling of fear and anxiety that her parents might not return. They wanted her to be strong and grown-up, because they knew nothing of vulnerability and it served them to have her strong. When she cried and was upset, they became angry. They told her that she was the oldest and that they expected her to behave like a grown-up and take care of things when they were not there. Tears and vulnerability brought pain, the pain of their disapproval. In addition, her parents told her that she was being selfish when she cried and was only thinking of herself. She had to think of her brother and be responsible for him. Being selfish was a very bad thing.

By the age of three or four, Mary had learned her lesson well, and she began to take care of her brother and the baby-sitters *and* her parents. She began to nurture everyone in her world, and she increasingly negated any behavior or impulse in herself that might be construed as selfish. In this way she handled the anxiety and fear of the vulnerable little girl who had been there before. By identifying herself with the primary-self system of giving and caring, she made a place for herself in the world and she was safe, to the extent that anyone is safe in a difficult family setting. Her disowned selves were her selfishness, which would have given her the ability to put herself first, and her vulnerability. Her own vulnerability remained totally neglected because caring for other people took priority. She always put herself last.

Mary had a daughter named Beth. Mary felt that Beth was a selfish child from the very beginning of her life. As far as Mary was concerned, Beth always seemed to put herself first, and the older she got, the more extreme she became in her behavior. She would take things from her mother's wardrobe and jewelry box and use them without ever asking for permission. She borrowed things from her brother and sister as well. She never helped around the house, and she left things a mess wherever she went. In every conceivable way, she became more and more of an opposite to her mother, and Mary could never understand what she had done wrong to bring this about.

For years Beth grew up with the judgments of her mother ringing in her ears: "You're selfish! You only think of yourself! The trouble with you is that you never think of anyone but yourself!" We are describing a common family interaction. Initially Beth may simply have been a spirited youngster who didn't like to share her toys with her younger siblings. Since Mary considered this unacceptable behavior, she judged Beth as selfish. Generally, a child either respects this judgment and tries to be unselfish or rebels against it and becomes increasingly the opposite of the judging parent. Beth went into rebellion, and from her earliest years she began to battle her mother's requirements that she be the giving and unselfish person that her mother was. It was a family at war, the opposing armies being the primary self of the mother (her giving nature) and the primary self of the daughter (her taking nature).

Imagine the long-term effect of Mary's judgments on Beth's Inner Critic. Beth may ultimately leave home in a major rebellion against her parents, but she will not leave her Inner Critic behind. Our Inner Critics do not remain at home when we go out into the big, wide world to get away from our judgmental families. They follow us everlastingly wherever we go—into our jobs, marriages, friendships, and ultimately into the parenting of our own children.

Since we all have primary selves and disowned selves, there is no way to avoid these kinds of interactions. Judgment is a way of life in human relationship and particularly in parent-child interactions because the disowned selves must be kept at bay. They are dangerous.

The selfishness of her daughter felt evil to Mary. It is often the case that the person we judge carries the feeling or quality of evil for us. Mary's feeling of evil about her daughter's behavior got transmitted into the core of the daughter's Inner Critic, making the Critic seem to possess the power of absolute judgment. The healing in this common kind of family pattern comes as Mary is able to claim her long-lost selfishness and the daughter is able to claim her long-lost giving and supportive nature. Mary and Beth are teachers for each other once they can reach beyond the pattern of judgment and self-criticism.

THE POWER FATHER

Jack is a powerful father. He was an athlete in school and continued his interest in athletics into his middle years. He became a successful businessman and he worships power and success and in particular "being out there" in the world. His son, Robert, is the exact opposite. Jack's attempts to make Robert into a physical child were always met with resistance and fear. Jack thought his son was a sissy, a baby, a crybaby. Robert was, in fact, a highly introverted and sensitive youngster who loved to play alone and make up stories. The constant judgment of his father threw him into a more extreme identification with his primary-self system, and he became contemptuous and rejecting of his father's value structures. With his own children, many years later, he demeaned physical prowess, so it should come as no surprise that one of his children was polarized in the direction of becoming a sports enthusiast. Such is the way of primary and disowned selves. Sometimes these judgments are expressed very directly, and sometimes they are held inside as silent judgments. As far as the Inner Critic is concerned, it really does not matter, and both provide good nourishment for it.

Robert's Inner Critic is fattened by the ongoing judgments of his father. Years later he is a successful attorney, but he never feels quite right about himself. He always compares himself to other attorneys, to other professionals. He is gnawed by self-doubt and feelings of unworthiness. No amount of support by his wife can change the way he feels. As the disowned self of his father, Robert suffers from the years of disparagement, and he will continue to be victim to the Inner Critic until the time comes when he becomes aware of it and begins to separate from it. He can work on the relationship to his father forever and ever, but the Inner Critic will remain untouched until he turns his attention inward.

Parents often ask us, "How can I help my child?" Our answer is very simple. *Shift your priorities. Discover what value structure you are identified with and separate from it. Then you will be in a position to claim your own disowned selves and your children will not have to carry them for you!*

IDENTIFYING WITH THE POWER PARENT

A child may carry the disowned self of the father, and the result is the kind of polarization that we have seen above. Or a child may identify with a power parent and disown the same vulnerable, sensitive self that the power parent disowns. June is strongly identified with her father, who is a very successful businessperson. Vulnerability is not to his liking, and he long ago lost contact with his creative and soul juices. June's mother carried the other side, as so often happens in marriages, and ultimately there was a divorce. In her younger years, June was very much identified with her mother. From high school on, however, the primary selves of power and success began to drive her personality, and from this new personality she became rejecting and judgmental of her mother. From the mother's standpoint, talking to June was like talking to her exhusband. The same judging quality appeared in June's voice, and a natural estrangement began to occur between mother and daughter.

June and her mother have pushed off in opposite directions, and they are carrying each other's disowned selves. The mother never dealt with her stronger impersonal and business energies in the marriage, and now she cannot deal with them with her daughter. From her primary self, which she would see as soft and feminine, she judges June's business identification and tells her she is just like her father. From her business and impersonal primary selves, June judges her mother's flowing softness and sees her as ineffectual in the world.

Deep within, the mother's Inner Critic repeatedly tells her how soft she is and how she has no business ability and no sense with money. The daughter's Critic constantly scolds her for being too harsh, selfish, demanding, and materialistic. Their mutual judgments of each other are so strong that they never are able to even become aware of the Inner Critic and how it is operating within each of them. The father is not at all aware of having an Inner Critic, which is common with people identified with power. He is living out of the fixed primary-self system of the successful, power-oriented businessman, and from this place he judges anything or anyone that does not conform to the standards of this self. Thus he completely adheres to this system and handles his vulnerability by judging other people rather than by listening to his Critic judge him. When such a person is ready to allow the inner dialogue to open up, you may be sure that the Critic is present, waiting to be heard. We might well give these Critics the special title of "Critics in Waiting." Usually only a crisis of some kind, such as serious illness, divorce, or a major business setback, will ignite the vulnerability of Critics in Waiting.

MARIE AS SOUL CHILD TO THE FATHER

Marie grows up in a family in which she is the soul child to the father. He is a creative, sensitive, and feeling man, and his needs are not met in his marriage. He does nothing to meet this issue with his wife, and, as is so often the case, he looks to his daughter to fill his soul needs. The mother is a very practical, down-to-earth woman, and both Marie and her husband are disowned selves for her.

As the years pass, however, this becomes a more serious issue because Marie and her father become closer. Out of the mother's own feeling of abandonment and loss, all quite unconscious, she begins to turn increasingly judgmental toward Marie. She attacks Marie for being a dreamer, for not playing outside with friends, for not being focused, for everything that she, the mother, is not. She never deals with the real issue in her life, which is the absence of a dynamic and loving connection to her husband plus the total rejection of her own introverted, soul nature.

Marie will be affected in many different ways by this kind of family dynamic. Our concern here is the development of her Inner Critic. It becomes very powerful, and it tends to paralyze her in her life. It sounds very much like her mother. Marie hates her mother for being judgmental toward her. She sees her father as always positive and loving. From our vantage point we can see, however, that her father's inability to deal with the marital issues left the mother out in the cold and helped to create the environment for her heavily judgmental attitude. It is obviously a source of real difficulty for a youngster to be split between a loving parent and a rejecting parent.

Much is being written and taught today on the issue of physical and sexual abuse toward children. Years of judgment by parents toward children who carry their disowned selves is another powerful kind of abuse. The Inner Critic that results from all this continues the abusive behavior. Until we are able to separate from this Inner Critic, the pattern of abuse goes on forever as the cycle of Judgment/Critic/Judgment spins on forever.

BUSINESS CHILD IN A SPIRITUAL FAMILY

Mel grows up in a family with strong spiritual values. His father is moderately successful in the world, but his belief system emphasizes love and spiritual development rather than success in the world. Mel is his total opposite. He has always loved money, and the older he gets, the more materialistic he becomes. His father and mother do not feel good about his materialistic emphasis, but their spiritual background requires them not to have judgments, which, in their belief system, are something to be avoided. As we have mentioned, the Inner Critic picks up these unspoken judgments, and they often carry much more power and authority than do the spoken ones.

Mel's Inner Critic becomes stronger as he grows older. It constantly tells him that he is not nice, that he is too materialistic, and that he does not have ethical social values. Everything that was being played out in his parents' heads becomes the Inner Critic symphony of his adult life. He tries very hard to separate from the perceived criticism of his real parents and thinks he has a handle on the problem. But without knowledge of the inner reality, without knowledge of the Inner Critic symphony, he will remain victim to the bad feelings it engenders.

SPIRITUAL CHILD IN A NONSPIRITUAL FAMILY

A large number of spiritually oriented people today were raised in families that had no interest in these matters. Vicki was a very sensitive, naturally spiritual, and psychically attuned child who found at a young age that she could pick up people's thoughts and feelings. When she communicated these out loud a few times, particularly in front of company, she was forbidden to do this anymore. She was told to get real and be like other children. She was taken to sporting events and forced to take all kinds of lessons that she did not want to take.

Her parents were obviously terrified of her psychic abilities. Anything having to do with dreams and mystery and intuition had to be squelched in their daughter because this was the only way it could be squelched in them. This is how children grow up against their natures. Vicki had to develop a primary-self system that colluded with her parents'; otherwise she would have been totally rejected by them. Her deep psychic and spiritual nature went underground, and she became a "grounded" person. Her Inner Critic was always attacking her for being too dreamy and unfocused because, try as she might, she could not stop her daydreaming and her fantasy process. The Critic, naturally, in its attempt to keep her safe, became the inner parent and constantly reminded her of the need to be here in the world and not try to leave it all the time. It remembered the pain of the little girl who was always being criticized, and in its attempt to protect her it criticized her more harshly than did her own parents.

THE EFFECT OF GROUPS TO WHICH WE BELONG

The faculty of any school that we attend is going to greatly affect the development of the Inner Critic. In English boarding schools, for instance, the primary-self system among faculty and students emphasizes "keeping a stiff upper lip." This refers to the need to stay in control, not cry, and not give in to feelings and emotions. As this primary-self system is adopted by the students, the Inner Critic will begin to attack them whenever they show or even begin to experience any kind of feelings. Since feelings become a kind of pariah in this situation, the students are vulnerable to the judgments of their schoolmates and the faculty.

In a school with a strong religious background, the primary-self system may have strong ideas about what behavior, thought, or feeling is appropriate and what is not appropriate. Let us say there is a code of honor about cheating. The Inner Critic will grab hold of this, and any thought or fantasy about cheating will be met with an attack on us. The Critic will be very active in seeing to it that we do nothing wrong in this regard. Whatever the rights and wrongs of the religious system, the Critic will attack us to make sure that we are doing the right thing.

The formal organizational structure that someone belongs to, such as a church or lodge, also has its own set of rules. People raised in a strong Catholic, Jewish, or Protestant background are given a set of injunctions about the way that they should act in the world. Their Rule Makers pick this up, and their Critics enforce the rules. Even when someone has totally rejected the value structure of the religion of his or her youth, the Inner Critic often continues to echo its teachings. Individuals who act out their freedom with the greatest abandon may have very strong Inner Fundamentalists. Otherwise they would not have to worship freedom so much. Real freedom does not mean doing what you want to do all the time. Real freedom means being able to embrace the Inner Conservative on the one side and the Free Spirit on the other side. *Real freedom emerges from the sweat, strength, and empowerment that comes from holding the tension of the many opposites that make up the human psyche.*

It is therefore important to remember that in all of our personal relationships and in all of our organizational connections we are dealing with the primary-self system of others. Where our primary-self system agrees with the outer one, there is no overt problem. We can identify with the system and disown what the person or system disowns. Where we are living out the disowned self of the outer person or organization, then we are subject to the judgment of the person or group. These judgments, over time, begin to fatten our Inner Critic. Even when we fight them on the outside, our Inner Critic is still growing because it has such a deep anxiety about being accepted and about our doing the right thing. Recognizing these outer judgments and learning to understand how we are constantly living out the disowned selves of other people can help us separate from their judgments and move through the maze of negative energy that exists in so many relational environments. Now let us look at some additional ways of dealing with your Inner Critic's reactions to the judgments of others.

BREAKING THE POWER OF "WHAT WILL PEOPLE THINK?"

Your Inner Critic is so terrified at the thought of the judgments of others that it never considers that, indeed, they may have none. As an Aware Ego, you have the option of deciding just how important the reactions of others are. You have a choice. Maybe it is important to take these reactions into consideration. For instance, we (Hal and Sidra) might want to dress more professionally when we present information in a formal lecture to a professional audience on the East Coast than we would when we are presenting to an informal group on the West Coast. This seems to be an important time to tune in to what others might think of us. But if we always dressed in terms of what people will think, we might never be truly comfortable or able to evolve our own individual style. We would try to be what we think they want rather than who we are.

Practice making this choice for yourself. Listen for the next time your Inner Critic says, "But what will people think?" Stop! Pay attention! What is it that your Inner Critic is afraid they will think? What is it afraid will happen if they do think this? Take a moment and consider just how important the reactions of others are in this situation. You might remind yourself that people often simply do not care. They are usually quite busy enough with their own lives and problems, thank you.

Now that you have considered how other people might react to you and the probable consequences of these reactions, move on to the other important aspect of this decision making. What is it that *you* want? What would be the best thing for *you* to do in this situation? What feels most comfortable or natural to *you*? Now make a real choice that includes *both* sets of considerations.

WHAT IF IT REALLY DIDN'T MATTER?

The Critic's famous "what will people think" question plagues many of us and keeps us behaving in ways that we think are acceptable and safe. It is important to have some awareness of the impact of our behavior on others, but the Critic's tyranny in this area is often absolute.

How about thinking of another statement, "What if it really didn't matter?" You might even do a "reality check," asking the other person how important something is to him or her. For instance, Janet is a very responsible, nurturing woman who thinks it is of the utmost importance to have a home-cooked meal ready each evening for her family. Although Janet works all day, she goes to a great deal of trouble to arrange the evening meals, even on those nights when she would rather not do so. She has never checked this out with her husband or her children, and her Inner Critic is merciless in its criticism of her if she ever skips an evening. One day she asks her family if they really care about home-cooked meals every night, and they surprise her by suggesting that it would be wonderful for all of them to go out a few times a week for something inexpensive and less formal. This would give her some time off and them a special treat. Like Janet, many of us probably take for granted that something that matters to us or to our primary selves is equally important to others. How about checking out to see if this is true? You may be surprised that many times it really does not matter.

Next, let us try something different. Think of what it would be like to be totally free of the injunction "What will people think?" Take a fresh piece of paper and write in a color that you do not ordinarily use (perhaps red or purple), "If it really didn't matter to anyone, I'd _____." Just play with it. This is not an agenda for changing your life! This is just a chance to play with some new ideas and see how you might possibly do things differently if you were not so worried about the impact of your actions on others and the repercussions in your relationships.

◆ HOW DID YOUR INNER CRITIC TRY TO ADAPT TO OTHER PEOPLE?

1. In growing up, you probably had to become a certain way in order to please your parents or your siblings. What did you have to do in order to please them?

a. What behavior was demanded of you?

b. Did you do what they wanted, or did you rebel?

c. Did you have an assigned role in your family? How was it different than the role of your siblings?

2. How did your Inner Critic fatten up on the judgments of people close to you?

3. Do you have any sense of how you might have played out the disowned self of your parent (or parents)?

4. Which of your teachers made you feel bad by their judgments, and which made you feel good by their lack of judgment toward you? What did you feel bad about?

Chapter Thirteen

The Incomparable Comparer

To compare ourselves to others greatly strengthens the authority of the Inner Critic. The Critic constantly replays events, reminding us where someone did something better than we did or how someone looked better than we did or how someone had greater poise and made a better impression than we could ever hope to make. It is indeed difficult for the creative juices to flow in the face of this barrage of comparison and negativity.

We have seen many different approaches that the Critic takes in its attempt to control our lives. One of the most effective methods it uses is to compare us to other people. This happens so automatically and naturally that it is difficult to catch hold of until we focus on the Critic and listen to the way it uses language. What we *feel* are bad feelings, depression, and a sense of general inadequacy. What we *hear* are the comparisons that the Critic is making behind the scenes.

The story begins in childhood in our family settings. Usually different children in a family have differing strengths and weaknesses. One child is feeling-oriented and another is a natural thinker. One child is very physical and another imaginative. One child is extraverted and another is introverted. These are natural differences that are, to a considerable extent, genetically based. As these children grow up, however, family and general environmental influences usually exaggerate the differences.

For example, John is an introverted and fantasy-oriented child. His older brother, quite the opposite, is extraverted, very much in the world and pragmatic in his approach to life. John feels vulnerable in relationship to his brother and his brother's strength in the world. His brother judges him for not being focused and for being weak. To make matters worse, John's parents value the personality of the brother much more than they value John's. This is where the Inner Critic comes in as the Incomparable Comparer. It constantly compares John to his brother. It always seems to be pointing out where he has fallen short and how well his brother has succeeded. Every family gathering is humiliating for John because his Critic goes into action a week before the event to start reminding him of his inadequacies.

Nor does the matter stop there. Since his brother carries many of his disowned selves, as John separates from his family and moves into his adult life, his Critic will be comparing him to every extraverted, successful man that he meets. These comparisons will go on endlessly. His wife may be very loving toward him and may well try to show him what a wonderful person he is and how his traits are to be valued. But his Inner Critic will have none of this. It behaves like a suit of armor and allows nothing positive to touch John. John will feel deeply jealous of men who are like his brother, and he will be wounded whenever he sees his wife talking in an animated way with men of this kind. Interestingly enough, the attractions and affairs that happen in relationship are often with someone who carries the disowned self of the wounded party.

As we have pointed out before, the Critic and Judge are two sides of a coin. John will no doubt judge his brother and people like his brother. It is entirely possible that he will be quite arrogant in these judgments. When the Inner Critic is strong, these judgments are often unspoken. The bottom line, however, will be John's sense that he is a victim to his brother. This is often a central factor in bringing about major breakups in family relationships. We cannot bear to live with these comparisons at close range, and ultimately we have to remove ourselves from the pain.

A young boy comes home from school with a D on his report card. His mother is upset by this and feels very vulnerable. Not being aware of or having a separation from her vulnerability, she is going to be taken over either by her Critic, her Judgmental Self, or both. What actually happens to this mother is that she feels inadequate. Her Inner Critic tells her that she has failed as a mother. To handle the pain of her Critic's remarks, she shifts into the Judgmental Self and says to her son, "Your brother never used to get grades like that." These comparisons of one child to another are very common in parent-child interactions. They prepare the Critic for its role as the Incomparable Comparer.

It is important to realize how much of this kind of comparing by parents comes from their own sense of inadequacy and vulnerability about a particular issue. Parents are constantly scolded by the voice of the Inner Critic, which tells them that they have not done or are not doing a good job parenting. A child gets into trouble of some kind or does poorly in school, and the first thing that the father and mother experience is the Inner Critic telling them it was *their* fault and making them feel terrible. The Inner Critic combines with the "what will people think" voice that gets worried if the child does not perform well. The sense of victimization and vulnerability that parents experience from this "what will people think" voice causes a great deal of pain and anguish in them. Jumping into the next step of making judgments and comparisons becomes a natural way of handling the situation. "Why must you get into trouble all the time? No one else ever did that! Just wait until you grow up and have a child like yourself! I just don't understand how you can lie like that. No one else ever behaved that way!" The Inner Critic/Comparer of the child takes in these statements and then uses them regularly to compare the youngster to the good boys and girls of the world who never get into trouble. These are painful comparisons, and life becomes an ongoing contest in which you lose most of the time.

SOME EXAMPLES OF THE INCOMPARABLE COMPARER

Here are some examples, taken from Voice Dialogue conversations, of the Inner Critic acting as the Incomparable Comparer:

Look how thin she is! I wish you would lose weight.

He made such a beautiful presentation.

She is so patient with her children.

That was such a brilliant interpretation! (Comparison implied.)

See how he is looking at her breasts. Men never look at your breasts that way.

He knows so much about so many things. Why don't you read more?

She has all kinds of friends. You have a real problem attracting people to you.

You are so selfish next to her. She is really there for people.

They are all more successful than you are.

Keep in mind, as we have pointed out, that the Comparer plays off our disowned selves. For example, if we tend to be more introverted and a friend is more extraverted, then the Critic will say something like, "She's so popular. You really need to get out more." Or if we know someone who is calm, peaceful, spiritual, and loving, the Critic might say, "You're always sticking your foot in your mouth. I wish you could be more like James. He's always so calm and controlled." This is happening in our friendships constantly, even with our very best friends.

VOICE DIALOGUE WITH THE INCOMPARABLE COMPARER

Ed has a very successful business and an equally successful Critic. Listen to it in this conversation as it uses the tool of comparison.

FACILITATOR (to Critic): It sounds as though you have a lot of control over Ed's life. He appears to be quite successful, but to hear him talk about himself one would think he's a total failure.

CRITIC: Well, you may think that he's successful, but the fact is that his brother is ten times wealthier than he is. And his brother is a lawyer also. So I wouldn't call him successful.

FACILITATOR: It sounds as though he's forever in his brother's shadow as far as you're concerned.

CRITIC: Well yes, but it isn't just his brother. His best friend has twice as much money as he does. He's a very bad manager. He's just not a businessman.

FACILITATOR: Could he learn how to be a more successful businessman? Could he ever be more effective so that you would be happy with him?

CRITIC: Look, I have to tell you, the guy's a loser. He always comes out on the bottom with the people that count. He just isn't a big player, and that's never going to change. It's like a curse.

FACILITATOR: You're pretty harsh with him, aren't you?

CRITIC: I'm not harsh, just truthful. He can't compete in the world with the big boys, and I just point that out to him and show him who these big boys are.

Ed's Critic is certainly a heavyweight Comparer. The early childhood years were particularly painful for him because his older brother, who was outgoing and successful at everything he tried, was the special son of both his parents. Having his brother be the special favorite of his parents, and hearing their constant overt and covert references to his brother's success, as well as Ed's own early worship of his brother, provided his Inner Critic with vast quantities of food, and it grew big and fat and quite out of control. When a sibling or friend or parent is particularly successful or special, the Critic/Comparer usually becomes extra powerful.

Let us look at this for a moment from the vantage point of Ed's brother. Even if his Critic/Comparer finds him superior to everyone else, his position in life is no more secure than if he were found inferior, because his Critic/Comparer is also too strong. If the Critic/Comparer operates with too much power and your worth as a human being depends upon being better than everyone else, then you become worthless when you are no longer the best!

Often the Critic will compare us to people that we do not know personally at all. For example, with very spiritual people, the Rule Maker will often set up some religious figure such as Jesus Christ or the Buddha as the model by which we should live. If we identify with this idea and try to be like Christ or Buddha in our behavior, then our Comparer has a real field day because any ill will or lack of perfection, by the standards of the Inner Critic, will be criticized and our gaze will constantly be brought back to the model of the life of the saint. Being compared to a saint, and with a rule in our minds that we must have ultimate enlightenment, the Critic literally evaluates everything we do in terms of whether it is moving us toward that enlightenment and whether our behavior is, in fact, like that of a saint. Since our home is the earth, and since we all have to live in society and earn a living, such comparisons are impossible to live up to and in fact can be quite crippling to our ability to function effectively in the world.

The Inner Critic might compare us to anyone—to a movie star or a business executive or a gas station attendant. If you do not do anything at all for your body and you happen to meet a real physical jock pumping gas, you may be sure that your Critic/Comparer will remind you of the glorious shape he is in and the miserable shape that you are in. This comparison can go on for weeks and months or even years. It is sad, but amusing too, to listen to an Inner Critic comparing you unfavorably to a person and event that took place five years or twenty years earlier in your life.

The Inner Critic uses siblings, parents, friends, colleagues, anyone it can think of to establish these comparisons. It requires a great deal of awareness and authority to get out from under this kind of attack. Think about your own life for a moment and think of who the Inner Critic uses as comparison models for you. Are they family members? friends? acquaintances? people that you do not know personally at all? It is only by becoming aware of these comparisons that you can separate from the Critic and begin to give it the help it needs. These comparisons are a significant part of the regular network programming of radio station KRAZY.

"THE ONLY WAY TO WIN IS NOT TO PLAY THE GAME"

In its role as the Incomparable Comparer, the Inner Critic is constantly putting you down. When you feel yourself sinking down into inadequacy as your Critic compares you to someone else, you can ultimately learn how to refuse to play the game. Next time this happens, start to say no firmly. It may take awhile, and we can assure you that the Critic as Comparer will reemerge from time to time, but you can gradually remove yourself from this part of the Critic's power by just refusing to listen to it.

It is also important to say no when a power voice wants to compare you favorably to others. These comparisons can be very seductive, but this game is as dangerous as the other! They are two sides of a coin. If your self-esteem is based on a power self that judges other people and that sees you as smarter or more successful or more attractive than they are, then you must always be the best. If you are not the best, then you are nothing and your Critic becomes terrified. It then works twice as hard, trying to move you back into a position of superiority by a new barrage of comparisons and criticisms.

The world of self-criticism on the one side and judgment toward others on the other side represents a major part of the dance of life. Hearing these voices, learning about their underlying vulnerability, and developing an Aware Ego in relationship to them gives us the ability to separate from them and to get off the dance floor when the wrong music is playing. The only way to win the game of judgment and self-criticism is to learn how not to play the game.

♦ HOW DOES THE INCOMPARABLE COMPARER
WORK IN YOUR LIFE?

1. Can you think of people in your life that the Inner Critic
compares you to? Does it compare you to one or more of your
siblings, cousins, parents, stepbrothers or stepsisters, colleagues,
or friends?

2. Pay close attention to what the Critic finds wanting in
you and how it uses these judgments in the comparisons that it
makes.

3. Does it compare you to public figures—people in the
world of film or politics or any other field of work?

4. What does the Incomparable Comparer say about your
body when it compares you with someone else?

5. As you listen to the Incomparable Comparer make its
comparisons, is there anything that you could do that could possibly make it right? Is there anything you could do that could
possibly make you equal to the other person? The answer to this
question is invariably a resounding "no!" We can only feel bad
until we recognize that these comparisons are being made by the
Critic and that we do not have to play the game.

_____

Chapter Fourteen

How the Inner Critic Sabotages
Our Relationships

*The Inner Critic makes each of us a child. As we become the
child in our relationships, we lose our sense of self. We are no
longer self-contained, self-respecting adults. We look to others for
validation. Our self-worth is based upon their opinions of us.
Thus, everyone around us becomes a mother or a father whose
support and approval is desperately needed to protect us from the
constant criticism of the Inner Critic.*

Through many devices the Inner Critic actively sabotages our
relationships. Just stop for a moment to think about the energy
drain caused by a hyperactive Critic. There is almost nothing left
over for our outside relationships once our Critic is through
with us. Much of our energy is spent in responding to its criticisms, either defending ourselves or feeling hopeless. Many of us
have relationships that are like this—our basic attention goes to
the Inner Critic rather than to the other person. After all, how
can you relate intimately to another person when you have a
Critic on your back with a choke hold around your neck?

Now let us consider the specific ways in which the Inner
Critic can make relationships miserable. Remember that the
Critic was born in relationship and that in its actions it often
recreates the original relationships we knew as a child. So the
first aspect we will consider is how our new relationships mirror the old.

THE INNER CRITIC AS RE-CREATOR OF OUR
CHILDHOOD RELATIONSHIPS

Our role in relationship is usually similar to the role that we played in our family of origin. In families, there is usually a division between the family members who have strong Inner Critics and those who have strong Judges. Thus, as we saw in chapter 12, certain family members will judge, while other family members have Inner Critics who pick up these judgments and use them; some family members are quick to assign blame, and others will readily accept it.

Jeri's father is a judgmental man who is constantly commenting on the shortcomings of others. Jeri develops a strong Inner Critic who picks up her father's judgments and uses them against her. Underneath it all, her Critic is hoping to make Jeri so perfect that her father will stop pointing out her shortcomings and will love her. But Jeri's role has been established; she is a victim to the judgments of the others in her family. Her Inner Critic has grown to enormous proportions. This makes her an instant victim to people in the outside world as well. If her husband tells her she is a fool, the Inner Critic agrees and Jeri believes him. If her children blame her for their own poor school performance and tell her that it was because she did not help them enough, her Critic agrees and she feels guilty. Jeri has become a guilt machine, and it is the Inner Critic who keeps starting the engine.

Conversely, Tom's mother had a strong Inner Critic. In response to her willingness to accept blame and to be the underdog, Tom became the judge in their relationship. He was quick to point out everything that she did wrong, from the way she took care of herself physically to her inability to deal powerfully in the world. He teased her, judged her, and generally blamed her for anything that went wrong in the family. So Tom developed a strong Judge rather than a strong Inner Critic. He, then, with his Judge as a primary self, recreates this original family situation in his current family.

Now let us imagine that Tom and Jeri team up in their lives. What scenario can we expect? Tom will become more and more judgmental toward Jeri. Her own Inner Critic will continue to grow until it matches that of his mother. She, in turn, has been drawn to Tom, a man with a strong Judge, because in her family of origin she was the one with the strong Inner Critic. Eventually Tom's Judge will match that of her father, as she keeps feeding it with her victim/daughter psychology.

Sometimes, however, when there is a particularly strong outer Judge, the Inner Critic will retire for a while and allow the outer Judge to take over its duties. Hal remembers talking to the Inner Critic of a woman who had been married to a very judgmental husband for many years. Her Inner Critic had this to say: "I went into retirement when she married Al. He did a great job. He criticized her all the time and I didn't have anything to do. I'm back now that they're divorced. And the truth of the matter is that I haven't forgotten any of my old tricks!"

It is important to note again that the Inner Critic and the Judge (the part of us who judges others) are two sides of the same coin. They are similar in the feelings that they carry and in the observations that they make. The only difference is that one judges us and the other judges the world. A strong Inner Critic, like the one that Jeri has, is a primary self and is often accompanied by an equally strong Judge who operates in silence. Thus Jeri is filled with silent judgments toward her parents and husband. There is as much passion in these silent judgments as in her self criticism. It is just that the judgments are held in silence.

It is a truism of relationship that every unspoken feeling or reaction toward another person can easily become a silent judgment. The other person senses these judgments and does not know why he or she is feeling uncomfortable, and possibly vulnerable, when seemingly in a position of clear superiority. Sometimes these judgments come out in the form of joking comments, sometimes they are spoken aloud to friends or to children, and sometimes they burst out under the influence of alcohol or at a time when anger breaks through the control system. Sometimes they are held in for fifteen or twenty years until the partner who is carrying these silent judgments, apparently without warning, files for divorce. These unspoken judgments can destroy the intimacy in our relationships. Last, but not least, they always work to strengthen the Inner Critic of the other person.

Just as a strong Inner Critic does not guarantee that no outer Judge is operating, so too the appearance of strength given by a strong Judge, as a primary self, does not necessarily mean that there is no Critic within. The outer Judge can silence an Inner Critic when someone is clearly a "winner" and in complete control. The Judge then maintains this position of ascendancy by being better than everyone else. However, when this position of superiority is threatened by a sudden reversal in fortune such as in illness, loss of job, retirement, or divorce, we often find that the Inner Critic goes to work.

Bad economic conditions will always activate many more Inner Critics. All the judgments that have been directed outward now move inward and attack, making these apparently strong people extremely vulnerable. After all, their power depended upon their perception that they were better than everyone else. That is one of the reasons why "powerful" judgmental men, such as Tom or Jeri's father, can become extremely vulnerable when the balance of power is upset and they are no longer clearly in control.

The role of the Inner Critic in maintaining our vulnerability is extremely important in all our relationships, so to this we next direct our attention.

THE INNER CRITIC TRIGGERS OUR VULNERABILITY

When we are vulnerable and unable to deal with our vulnerability, we cannot relate properly to another human being, whether this relationship is romantic, familial, a friendship, or work related.

The existence of a normally active and moderately well-nourished Inner Critic plays a major role in keeping us vulnerable. The Inner Critic and its constant complaints about us and the way in which we live makes us feel inadequate because, when it is operating and we are not aware of it, we just cannot seem to do enough or be good enough so that we can feel good about ourselves.

For instance, if we give a big workshop and it basically goes well, Sidra's Inner Critic may have noticed that someone in the last row left early. With the Inner Critic commenting on this, she will feel vulnerable. Or if we choose to write this book but in so doing we must put off working on our scheduling, running errands, or making notes for our next teaching assignment, our Inner Critics have the opportunity to lecture us on our shortcomings and to make us vulnerable about what is not being done. No matter how much writing we do or how good it is the Inner Critics can tell us that we neglected our other work, our physical routines, each other, our families, etc., etc. (The etceteras are to show you that the Inner Critic does have a way of running on and on.)

Sandie is a working mother who has just driven her children to grade school and has gone on to her job. She likes her work and is looking forward to a productive day. She arrives at the office to find that her youngest child has left his lunch in the car. Her Inner Critic immediately begins to berate her about how and why she forgot the lunch. Depending on its level of sophistication, it might even criticize her lack of nurturance and caring as an indication that she is not adequately in touch with her deep femininity.

Sandie feels totally vulnerable and worried about the consequences of this trauma for her son. She is concerned about the judgments of her real mother, who thinks it is shameful for a woman to go to work while she still has school-age children. Sandie's mother does not even have to be present for these concerns to surface; the Inner Critic is repeating all her comments.

Now, rather than feeling self-assured and excited as she starts her day, Sandie feels vulnerable and will become a victim to just about any judgmental person in her vicinity. Her Inner Critic makes her see herself as deserving of their judgments and will be quick to point out to her that she has sabotaged her relationship both to her son and to her co-workers. She is in a state of complete vulnerability.

See how it works? No matter what you do or how you do it, it is just not good enough for your Inner Critic, and your Inner Child feels vulnerable and uncared for.

THE INNER CRITIC MAKES YOU A CHILD IN YOUR RELATIONSHIPS

When the Inner Child feels vulnerable and uncared for, and when you do not know how to parent it properly, it will look for parenting elsewhere. It will go elsewhere for reassurance and protection. Let us return to the workshop in which somebody leaves early and Sidra's Critic gets activated. When her Inner Critic starts to talk, her Inner Child feels dreadful. If Sidra has no Aware Ego operating, then she cannot be objective about this and deal with the Critic's complaints and her child's feeling of failure. The next step in this scenario is that her Inner Child will turn to Hal for reassurance, as though he were her father. We now have two grown-up people, who have just done a good piece of work together and who should feel good about themselves and each other, driven apart by the Inner Critic's attack. Hal must become father to Sidra's Inner Child. He can either be a good father and reassure her, or he can become irritated with her for her lack of objectivity and her feelings of inadequacy. But a father he will become.

This relationship of the parent part of one person (Hal) with the child part of another person (Sidra) is what we call a "bonding pattern." Bonding patterns are natural ways of relating to one another. When the "good" parent relates to the child, the pattern feels warm and safe; when the "bad" parent relates to the child, the pattern feels dreadful. In this example, if Hal's Good Father reassures Sidra's Inner Child, she will feel cared for and safe, at least for the moment. If Hal's Judgmental Father becomes irritated with her, her Inner Child bonds into this Judgmental Father and she will be miserable. When this happens, Sidra's Critic continues to chastise her on the inside and Hal's Judgmental Father matches these comments on the outside.

The Inner Critic, as we have said, activates the Inner Child and turns us into inadequate children. The Inner Child cannot help itself; it will seek out parenting. If we cannot protect it against the attacks of the Inner Critic, it will seek out another parent. When it finds another parent, it bonds with this parent and we become children in our relationship. This is not the way to care for the Inner Child properly. In the long run, nobody can take care of your Inner Child as well as you yourself can.

As you can see, the Inner Critic keeps us feeling insecure and childlike. When it is operating, we feel like children who have done something wrong and probably will never be able to do anything right. Let us look at some other examples of how the Inner Critic directly affects relationships by creating bonding patterns.

THE INNER CRITIC AND BONDING PATTERNS

Henry loves Betty. They have been dating for six months now, and he wants to do something special for their anniversary. He plans to surprise her; he decides to bring her flowers and to take her out to dinner at her favorite restaurant. He makes his preparations and is ready for the big evening. He is a bit nervous, but he ignores this.

Henry is a romantic. In this way, he is different from the rest of his family of origin. His father is a gruff, unromantic, judgmental man. He is critical of any feelings and particularly of anything that might suggest softness or vulnerability. Because his father is so judgmental, Henry has developed a strong Inner Critic. As Henry gets dressed for the evening, his Inner Critic (who sounds a good deal like his father) begins to tell him that the evening is not going to work. It says that he is being a fool, he is too romantic, women do not like men who treat them too well, women like men who are tough, they do not like softies.

By the time he is ready to meet Betty, Henry feels like a foolish child. He is awkward and has trouble thinking of something to say to her when, only hours earlier, he was full of exciting thoughts and feelings and a great deal of love and tenderness. Instead of a romantic man who is looking forward to being with his woman, Henry has become an uncomfortable awkward child who looks to Betty for appreciation and love but fears that she will find him inadequate, just as his Inner Critic does.

Although Betty previously has not thought of Henry as a child, she now sees him as one and reacts to him as a parent. For a time she may react as a "good" parent, praising him for what he has done for her. This is a bonding pattern, not a conscious interaction between two people. At some point, however, Betty finds herself becoming irritable with him and she turns into a "bad" parent. As Henry's Inner Critic criticizes him on the inside, she will begin to judge him from the outside, perhaps even repeating some of his Critic's criticisms about his being too soft and needy. This, then, re-creates the uncomfortable relationship that Henry had with his father. A truly miserable bonding pattern has been created.

For another example of the Inner Critic's influence on bonding patterns, let's look at Ethel and her children. Ethel's mother was not a very motherly type and Ethel did not really like her very much, so her Pusher and her Perfectionist have decided that she must be the perfect mother. Her Inner Critic is intent that she live up to their expectations. So Ethel reads magazine articles and books and tries to give her children the advantage of all the new information on child rearing. She knows the mistakes that her mother made with her, and she does not want to repeat them.

Ethel is basically a good mother. She is thoughtful about her relationship to her children and she truly loves them. But the catch is this: it is not Ethel who is in charge here, it is her Pusher and Perfectionist, and her Critic is always available to point out all the "mistakes." Her Critic will tell her that she is emotionally unavailable, that she is too available, that she should be planning more interesting and challenging activities for her children, that she is overscheduling them and not allowing them time for imaginative self-expression, that she is stressing academics too much, or that she is not helping them to get ahead in school like the other mothers who do homework with their children. Ethel can do little that is right, because there is always an opposite opinion on how to best raise children.

This makes Ethel completely vulnerable. She is actually in a child relationship to her children. She is in a bonding pattern with them. If they are "good" parents and love her and think that she has done a good job, she feels good; if they become "bad" parents and are angry with her, she is devastated. This makes it almost impossible for her to do anything that will make them unhappy. It is difficult for her to set limits, to ask them to do anything they do not want to do, or to correct them.

Because of her Critic's judgments on her child rearing, Ethel is a child to the children's teachers as well. She is in a bonding pattern with them, much as with her children. Ethel's Inner Child looks to the children's teachers for approval and validation. If they think that her children are well behaved, hardworking, and intelligent, she feels good about herself. If they say anything negative, she feels bad. Ethel is also a child when she is around the other mothers. Her Inner Critic, as the Incomparable Comparer, is quick to point out where other mothers do the job better, and she spends a good deal of time feeling inferior to them. If she has any interactions with these mothers, she will be in bonding patterns with them as well.

What you can see from all these examples is that *the Inner Critic makes each of us a child*. As we become the child in our relationships, we lose our sense of self. We are no longer self-contained, self-respecting adults. We look to others for validation. Our self-worth is based upon their opinions of us. Everyone around us becomes a mother or a father whose support and approval is desperately needed to protect us from the constant criticism of our Inner Critic. The irony in this is that nobody else can give us the approval we need. Nobody can give us anything but temporary relief from the pain caused by the Inner Critic. Only we can rescue ourselves from this ceaseless bombardment.

THE INNER CRITIC MAKES US UNRELIABLE AS PARTNERS OR FRIENDS

The Inner Critic's ability to make us unreliable partners and friends is slightly different from its power to make us children in relationship. As an equal partner, you must be reliable. *When your Inner Critic is active, you basically cannot be counted on as a competent, adult, objective partner, whether this partnership is at work or in a personal relationship.*

Your Critic can make you unreliable. With an active Inner Critic you cannot predictably and consistently define boundaries or stand up for yourself, your friends, family, or co-workers. An active Inner Critic leaves you vulnerable to the opinions and judgments of others. As we have shown, you become a child in relationship to the people around you. You need them to validate you. As a result of this, wherever you are, you are the child and you will react to the opinions and needs of others. You are likely to vacillate and change as others demand this of you or as they judge you.

The Inner Critic causes you to distrust yourself, and this too leaves you open to the influences of others. Let us see how this works. It is the week after Open School Night. The children's teachers have spoken to the parents about limiting TV watching because the children are not doing their homework. You and your wife decide to set limits with the children and enforce them. No TV until the homework is done! It is all very clear. Then your wife leaves to go to a meeting. Your Inner Critic begins to harass you over something you did at the office, and you start to feel vulnerable. Now when the children say, "Oh, Daddy, just let us watch a little TV and then we'll do our homework. Come on!" you simply cannot say no. Your Critic reminds you that you made a stupid decision earlier in the day, and you now begin to distrust this decision as well. It suggests to you that perhaps you did overreact to the teacher's demands. In addition to the fact that you no longer trust the decision that you made, you are feeling foolish and vulnerable and you want your children to love you. The children are not likely to show you much immediate affection if you insist that they do their homework!

On an inner level, your Critic is attacking you and you feel vulnerable; this has turned you into a child in relationship to your children. Now you need your children to "parent" you and to love you. So you let them watch TV even though you and your wife agreed that they should not. You have proven yourself an unreliable partner. Simple, isn't it? The Critic can undermine you when you are separated, and without realizing that you are doing so you betray your partner, leaving him (or her) vulnerable and, sooner or later, judgmental and angry.

The same pattern can happen at work. You run a business in which each person is expected to be responsible. Ernest has been slacking off, and you and your partner decide that it is your turn to talk to him about this. By the time you reach Ernest, your Critic has pointed out to you that you are so incompetent you have no right to discipline anyone. You no longer can speak firmly and objectively to Ernest. Instead, you are tentative and a little apologetic in what should have been a clear and objective definition of expectations. You have unintentionally betrayed your partner.

In a last example, a piece of work needs to be done. A report has to be written at work, a plumber needs to be called for the household, estimates must be obtained for an addition to the house, reservations have to be made for your group of friends for dinner at a restaurant of your choosing. You promise, with enthusiasm and the full intention of doing so, that you will take care of any one of these matters. Then, when you are alone, the Inner Critic attacks. It is sure that you will do this wrong. The report will be dreadful; the plumber will do a bad job and will probably overcharge you; you really do not know how to call for estimates and, besides, nobody will ever pay any attention to you because you do not command authority; nobody will like the restaurant you have chosen and they will all know that you are a boor. Even though you would like to do as you promised, you become paralyzed and cannot move ahead. You disappoint the others. They will probably feel betrayed and vulnerable and then become irritable with you.

THE INNER CRITIC ENERGETICALLY ELICITS THE JUDGE FROM OTHERS

The best way to avoid being judged by others is not to judge yourself. But with a reasonably active Inner Critic, this is just about impossible. The Critic literally activates the Judge in the people around us, even in those who usually are not very judgmental. As Hal is fond of saying, "A little white rabbit will become a stern and unforgiving judge when you have a strong Inner Critic."

Part of this is nonverbal, or energetic, if you will. The Inner Critic sets up a vibration like a tuning fork. Just as the tuning fork touched to a box brings forth a similar tone from the box, so does the Critic bring forth a similar tone from other people. If the tuning fork sings out the note A-sharp, then the box will also sing out an A-sharp. Just as there are Inner Critics everywhere, so also are there Judges just waiting to get their turns. As the Judges of the world sense the A-sharp of the Critic, they respond with their own A-sharp. What a miserable situation! The Inner Critic's worst nightmare comes true over and over again. The world is full of judgmental parents!

It is almost impossible to avoid this reaction. If someone is having a Critic Attack, it is almost impossible for the other person not to become judgmental. The guilty, victim child will draw out the judgmental, blaming parent from the people around him or her. Conversely, people who are judgmental will activate the Inner Critic in the other person with all the attendant feelings of inadequacy.

Most of you had the following experience as children: You did something wrong, you knew you had been bad, and you felt guilty. When your parents came into the room, they looked at you and saw that you looked guilty. Then they asked something like, "Now what have you been up to?" *As adults, our guilt feelings elicit the same kinds of accusations from the outside world that they did from our parents. It is not necessary for us to say anything aloud because our looks, our energies, and the signals that we are sending out are enough.*

THE INNER CRITIC ELICITS THE JUDGMENTS IN OTHERS

When we move to the level of verbal interaction, we can watch the Judge elicited by the comments of the Inner Critic. Emma is an attractive young woman, but she has a very active Inner Critic. Her Critic has decided that Emma's nose is all wrong and that she should have it fixed. Emma begins to ask her friends their opinions. Most of them think that her nose is just fine the way it is, and they tell her so. There is nothing objectively wrong with it. But then she continues and says, "Well, if I made it a little narrower here and a little shorter there, wouldn't it look good?" This brings forth the Judge in just about everyone, and at this point they are likely to agree with Emma's Critic that, yes, it would be a good idea to have her nose fixed.

Jane is a pretty woman with a lovely body, but she has a simply monstrous Inner Critic. She is obsessed with what is wrong with her body. She looks at her cellulite, she thinks that she is fat, she counts her wrinkles, she frets over how badly her clothes fit, she bemoans her lack of firmness, she compares herself unfavorably to other women. Her husband, Frank, used to think that she looked pretty good. But now, after listening to her talking about all the things that are wrong with her, he is beginning to wonder if maybe, after all, she is right. Over the years, Frank's judgments are elicited and he starts to look at Jane the way that her Inner Critic looks at her. Now Jane does not look too good to Frank either. Her Critic's worst fears have come true.

The Inner Critic can affect the evaluation of one's work as well. Charles hands his supervisor a report. It is a fine report, but Charles's Inner Critic does not think so. She (Charles's Critic is a she because it sounds just like his mother, who was a schoolteacher) has already shown him everything that is wrong with the report. For a few moments the supervisor does not say anything. Charles cannot bear the silence, and at the urging of his Critic he says, "Well, I know that the conclusions don't follow from the findings if you want to look at it in a truly rigorous fashion." The supervisor, who had not thought that at all, now picks up directly from Charles's Critic and begins to criticize the report and point out all the shortcomings that had not been important to him earlier. It is no longer the supervisor but the supervisor's Judge that is now on the job. Actually, the conclusions are fine, as is the report, but a good Critic working with a powerful Judge can make just about anything look bad, and that is what happens to Charles's report.

THE INNER CRITIC AS AN INTERPRETER OF SILENCE

The Inner Critic is basically a verbal self that cannot bear silence. This affects our relationships in two ways.

First of all, as we saw with Charles in the last example, the Critic rushes in to interpret the silence of others—disastrously! As Charles waited for his supervisor to comment upon his work, the Critic began to panic. As we have said earlier, the Inner Critic is basically terrified that we will be rejected, that we will be found not good enough. Now Charles knows very well that it takes awhile to read a report that someone else has spent two months in preparing. It will obviously take his supervisor some time to look over the report, digest its contents, and then evaluate it. But Charles's Inner Critic does not know about this; his Inner Critic hears the deafening silence and panics. The Inner Critic takes over, and since there is no Aware Ego, there is no one to remind Charles of the objective fact that this will take some time. Instead, his Critic feels unbearable pressure from its own interpretation of the silence and uncontrollably blurts out its criticisms of the report in an effort to please the supervisor.

Charles gives us one painful picture of how the Inner Critic handles the silence of another person. What do you think your Inner Critic is going to say when another person falls silent in your presence? If you are a woman, and a man that you have just met at a party suddenly stops speaking, is your Inner Critic likely to tell you that he has been struck dumb, that he has just been overwhelmed by his sexual feelings or by the thought of how much he wants you to like him? Not likely. Your Inner Critic is far more likely to tell you that he is bored or angry or that he wishes you would go away because he feels stuck with you and he wants to talk to someone else in the next room.

In intimate relationships, we do not usually keep talking all the time. If we do, it can get fairly exhausting. But the silence, again, is a threat to the verbal Critic. The Critic begins to worry, and it fills the silence with an internal monologue. It thinks of all sorts of reasons why the other person is disappointed, annoyed, or otherwise upset with us. It, of course, never thinks that the other person could be sleepy, thinking about lunch, worried about something at work, going over a list of things that have to be done, or involved with any of the thousands of matters that clutter up our minds. For the Inner Critic, this is seen as a silence that is filled with judgment and we, somehow, must have done something wrong. If you tune in carefully, you might even hear it say something like: "What did I do?" "Why is she (he) not talking to me?" "Why is he (she) looking so irritated?" "What's the matter?"

The second way in which the Critic's inability to tolerate silence affects our relationships is that it blocks intimacy directly by not allowing us to move into a "being" state. It keeps us in a "doing" mode. The being state is the one in which we can just be with another human being without having to perform. We can just relax together with no place to go and nothing to do. This is an intensely intimate way to be with another person. But this type of quiet panics the Critic, who must fill every space with doing something and with speech.

Now let us look further at the ways in which the Inner Critic blocks true intimacy in relationships.

THE INNER CRITIC BLOCKS INTIMACY IN RELATIONSHIPS

Because the ability just to be, silently, with another person is such an important aspect of intimacy, we would like to develop the last point more fully. The Inner Critic is panicked by silence and does not allow this being state. There is no opportunity, therefore, for the deep and peaceful intimacy of silence.

The Inner Child is one key ingredient for our truly intimate connections with others. This child brings a depth of feeling, a spontaneity, and a sensitivity in relating to all our close relationships. But when the Inner Child is badly abused by the Inner Critic, it is not available for relationship. It is too hurt and damaged to be able to emerge and connect with another human being. This, then, continues the cycle. The Critic maintains the abandonment and the inner abuse of the Inner Child by keeping it isolated from the love, intimacy, and support of others who might be able to help in its healing.

The Inner Critic keeps us victimized by its constant harangues. It tells us that we do not deserve anything good. Thus we often relate to others as a victim. This brings forth pity or judgment in others, not a sharing, admiring, and equal intimacy.

In an intimate, sexual relationship, an active Inner Critic kills Aphrodite (the goddess of love). It is a talker, not a lover. It has no real way of relating to another person in a sensual fashion. To make matters even worse, it has an unfortunate habit of criticizing you for the way you look and the way you perform. These particular criticisms tend to diminish sexual activity and performance. After all, if you are worried about what you look like, what you smell like, how you sound, if you are performing properly, if you are sexy enough, if you are as passionate as you should be, or if your orgasms are good enough, you are not very likely to enjoy your natural sexuality. Inner Critics tend to be experts when it comes to sexual performance.

In addition to all this, the Inner Critic can keep you from taking in anything good. Even though your friends or intimates may be positive in their comments to you, the Inner Critic has it in its power to nullify their love and praise. It may wait until you are alone later in the day or, better yet, until the wee hours of the morning before it reviews the nice things that others have said about you. Then, even though you would just love to believe them, it effectively blocks out their loving or complimentary remarks with comments like the following:

They really didn't mean that.

He just felt sorry for you, so he said something nice.

You just fooled them.

If she really knew what you were like underneath, like I do, she'd never say that.

Wait until he gets closer to you, then he'll find out what you're really like.

She's just saying what she knows you want to hear.

He just wants something from you.

It's a manipulation, she doesn't mean it.

There's a whole part of the story that they just don't know.

For some of us, the Inner Critic flips over to the other side and becomes the Judge and we distance ourselves from others. It happens when we really love somebody and we are particularly vulnerable in relationship. This is the signal for the Inner Critic to get worried. It starts to criticize us in order to make us perfect enough to deserve the other person, and then, when the pain or anxiety gets too great, it triggers our Inner Judge. The Critic disappears and the Judge takes over. We find ourselves pushing away from the other person because everything he or she does displeases or even disgusts us. When the Judge takes over suddenly in this way, it is often a good idea to go looking for the Critic who is likely to be operating underneath.

So when you are thinking about some of the difficulties that you encounter in your relationships, we suggest that you look to your friend, the Critic. Check it out, see what it has been doing, and you may discover that it has been playing a major—and all too familiar—role as an unintentional saboteur.

HOW CAN YOU PROTECT YOUR RELATIONSHIPS FROM YOUR INNER CRITIC?

As you look over the exercises at the end of this chapter, you will see how your Inner Critic can turn you into either an inadequate child or a judgmental parent in your relationships with others. These patterns, which we call bonding patterns, cause much unhappiness. Our book *Embracing Each Other* describes these bonding patterns in detail and tells about how to deal with them. In the present book, we are specifically concerned with the role played by the Inner Critic.

What can you do about these bonding patterns in your relationships? First of all, with the help of this book and all these exercises, become alert to the actions of your own Inner Critic, notice your own patterns of behavior, and begin to take steps to change them as suggested. You can use any system of growth or therapy to supplement our suggestions. Anything that helps you to separate from the Inner Critic and to assume your own authority in life will help in this. This is a gradual process. Your Inner Critic is not likely to disappear completely overnight, but with persistence you can diminish its power and transform the Critic so that you can use its unbelievable intelligence and boundless energy in more fully supportive ways.

The very best thing that you can do for your relationships is to be in tune with your own needs and feelings. Your Inner Critic comes into operation when you are vulnerable, and it fears for your safety. If you take charge and deal effectively, it does not need to do so. All psychospiritual work that you do is going to help to make you a more effective person, make you better able to take care of yourself, and thus reduce the anxiety level of the Critic. Another way of putting this is that if you care adequately for your own Inner Child, your Inner Critic can retire from its job as parent. When your Inner Critic is no longer tearing you to pieces, you will be able to relate to others with far greater satisfaction.

Remember that your Inner Critic will activate the Judge in others. Do not make a habit of repeating its criticisms to someone whose love and admiration you want! If you do, you will just be drawing attention to your own shortcomings, whether they are real or imagined, and you will be inviting judgments. Deal with your Critic's comments in settings that are specifically designed for this (like your support groups or in psychotherapy), but not in your everyday interactions with people whose relationships you value.

If someone is silent in your presence and you begin to feel very uncomfortable, take a moment to remember that your discomfort is probably a reaction to your Inner Critic's unspoken interpretation of the silence. Check your thoughts as we suggest in exercise 8 at the end of this chapter. What do you think the other person is thinking? Now, try a reality check. Ask the other person what he (or she) is thinking. You may be surprised at the answer. The answer may truly be "nothing," because many people spend time just sitting still with their minds blank. Or it may well be something that has nothing to do with you but is worrying the other person, like finances. It is only some of the time that you are being judged. These reality checks provide you with tangible information, and they help to calm the anxiety of your Inner Critic.

Last, but not least, look at the information from exercise 9 at the end of this chapter, and pay attention to what happens when someone says something nice to you. Then, when your Inner Critic begins to counter a compliment with its nasty comments, be aware that it is your Critic and not necessarily God who is speaking. As you realize that it is just your Inner Critic trying to protect you by shielding you, notice how it is keeping out the love or support of another, and experiment with removing the Critic's shield. See what it feels like to let the positive messages in. Of course, you must always be alert to the possibility of manipulation by others, but most of the time positive messages are just what they seem to be on the surface.

All in all, any work that you do separating from your Inner Critic will greatly improve your intimate relationships. It has long been a part of our folk wisdom that you cannot love others or be loved until you love yourself, and there is no way that you can truly love yourself until your Inner Critic is no longer in charge of your self-image.

◆ HOW DOES YOUR INNER CRITIC SABOTAGE
YOUR RELATIONSHIPS?

As we said at the beginning of this chapter, your Inner Critic evolved in your familial relationships and plays a part in your current relationships. These exercises will help you to see how this works.

1. In your family of origin, with which family members did you play the role of the Judge? What did you judge about them?

2. In your family of origin, do you remember which family members judged you? If so, what were their criticisms? (This may already have been answered in the exercises at the end of chapter 1.)

3. Can you hear your Inner Critic repeating these criticisms of you? If so, what are they? (This also may have been answered by the exercises at the end of chapter 1.)

4. Where, in your current relationships, do you sometimes become the Judge? Whom do you judge currently? Do you sense this other person's feelings of inadequacy? (This will be an indication of bonding patterns.)

5. Where do you sometimes feel like an inadequate child in your current relationships? (This will give you a clue as to where you are living in bonding patterns.)

6. Who in your present relationships seems to judge you? Whose judgments frighten you? What judgments are particularly upsetting?

7. Do you remember the last time that someone became silent in your presence? What did you think that person was thinking about you?

8. The next time that someone is silent in your presence, try to tune in to how your Inner Critic interprets this silence. Do you begin to think that the silent person is angry with you? disapproving of you? bored with you?

9. What does your Inner Critic whisper in your ear when someone says something nice to you?

Chapter Fifteen

In Summary

We have seen that the Inner Critic is a major player on the stage of relationship. Let us review some of the important ways in which it influences our style of relating.

Our Inner Critics are deeply concerned about our relationships with others. They:

worry a great deal about what others think of us;

are panicked by the thought of looking foolish;

are terrified that we might be judged, rejected, or abandoned;

evaluate our readiness for relationship and always find us inadequate;

are terrified that we will not be good mates or parents.

Our Inner Critics grow up in our family of origin. They:

echo the judgments of us that we heard from family members or other important people in our lives (e.g., you're selfish, bossy, stupid, weak);

echo our judgments of others, particularly our family members, warning us not to be like them (e.g., weak, passive, etc.);

judge our disowned selves as being unacceptable and dangerous;

are very righteous;

are supported by the family members or groups that helped them to develop in the first place;

compare us to everyone around and find us inferior.

The Inner Critic is a major saboteur in our relationships. It keeps us vulnerable and childlike and puts us at the mercy of the judgments, needs, and demands of everyone around us. It tells us we have no right to be separate, to have our own needs, to establish boundaries. In relationship, the Inner Critic:

re-creates our childhood relationships;

responds to the judgments of everyone around us by agreeing with them;

keeps us vulnerable;

causes us to play the role of child to the parent in others;

can cause us to distrust ourselves;

energetically activates the Judge in others;

directly elicits judgmental comments from others;

interprets silences as negative reactions of others toward us by asking us what it was that we did wrong;

interferes with our sexuality;

is overly verbal and cannot allow the silence and depth of being together that allows intimacy.

Last, but certainly not least, the Inner Critic prevents intimacy directly by shaming and abusing our Inner Child so that it cannot relate properly to others. It is this Child that carries our deepest sensitivities and feelings and is a major factor in truly intimate connections. When it is frightened, abused, and feels like a victim, it cannot relate normally and naturally, and the deep, soul-satisfying intimacy that it brings with it is missing from all our relationships.

FOUR

Transforming the
Inner Critic

Chapter Sixteen

Understanding the Underlying Anxiety of the Inner Critic

As we tune in to the Inner Critic, we begin to perceive it as an alarm system that signals a call for help. Someone is dialing 911. Someone is alerting us to the possibility of pain, shame, or abandonment. It is as though the Inner Critic cries, "Look out! Please help me because I cannot handle this situation!"

One of the fundamental principles of learning to work with and handle the Inner Critic is what we call the conversion principle. What we mean by this is the ability to convert your distress at the Critic's attack upon you to an understanding of the underlying anxiety and fear that motivates this attack. We have alluded to this idea many times in the course of this book. We now wish to bring a deeper focus to this issue and to teach you how to use this understanding in a practical way.

People respond in a variety of ways to the attack of the Inner Critic. Some people do not know what is happening and just feel depressed. In this case, they are victims of the Critic and of life in general. Others jump to the attack and, instead of feeling inadequate and depressed, become judgmental toward other people. A strong Judgmental Self is a sure sign that a strong Inner Critic is operating beneath the surface. As we have mentioned previously, it is often the case that people who appear the most powerful and judgmental are at their core intensely vulnerable and self-critical. Under the impact of some major adversity they may discover that their Inner Critics are, indeed, alive and well.

A third way of dealing with the Critic is to project it onto the people in one's life who tend to be judgmental. Here the battle seems to be with the people on the outside, and the Inner Critic is able to do its job with quiet authority and without interference on the inside. We find this often with people who have had very judgmental parents. They live life as rebellious children and project their Inner Critics onto the outer authorities of the world, who remind them of their judgmental parents. Similarly, some people may break from formal religions because the religious teachings seem too judgmental. These people often move in the opposite direction and adopt a value structure that is antithetical to everything that their church stood for in their earlier lives. Judgment remains projected onto the church where, indeed, it may reside. Unfortunately, such people may never realize that the church and its judgments also live inside their heads and that the judgments they so hate are directed toward themselves via the Inner Critic and toward the church and other people via their judgmental nature. The more extreme the judgments with which we were raised, the harder it is to step out of the family war zone and realize that it is all happening on the inside as well as the outside.

A fourth way of responding to Critic attacks is to turn around and attack the Inner Critic itself. People who do this usually have some sense of the Critic on an inner level. They will jump to the other side of what the Critic wants. For instance, if the Inner Critic says that Mamie is too self-absorbed and should be nicer to Aunt Em, Mamie gets angry and refuses to phone Aunt Em on her birthday. People like Mamie thus become rebellious sons and daughters to whatever it is that the Critic is advocating. This is reinforced, as we have seen above, by having a judgmental parent on the outside who is saying the same thing that the Critic is saying. Thus the individual is rebelling against both the outer parent figure and the demands of the Inner Critic.

People may also rebel against the Inner Critic if they have been in therapies where they were taught to assert themselves against its inner demands. They learn to be strong and tough, and they say to the Inner Critic in no uncertain terms, "You won't get away with this kind of crap anymore!" Their Inner Critics do not go away. They simply go underground and wait for another day, and they then reassert themselves as smugly and powerfully as ever. Attacking the Inner Critic solves nothing.

GOING UNDERNEATH THE CRITIC

What we are proposing is that the attack of the Inner Critic is in fact a cry for help. It is like an alarm system that rings inside of you, warning you of danger. It lets you know that, at some level, the Inner Critic is unhappy, anxious, and deeply concerned about what you are doing, feeling, or thinking. It fears that you will experience pain, rejection, or abandonment. Your Critic is terrified that you are going to look foolish and bring shame onto the system.

To go beneath the criticisms of the Inner Critic and convert your distress to understanding, you must always remember how and why the Critic was born. You must remember the important role that it has had to play in protecting that very young, vulnerable, unprotected, and sensitive child that you used to be and that continues to live within you today and forever.

The Critic remembers the pain you felt when your feelings were hurt. It remembers the humiliation and the shame that you experienced and how terrible that was. It remembers the hurt when people laughed at you, when your mother screamed at you in front of friends, when your father laughed at the wooden box that you made with your first tools. It will do anything to help you avoid that pain, even if it means destroying you. It remembers vividly the terror you experienced when you felt abandoned by your parents and siblings, whether this abandonment was physical or energetic. It remembers the anxious nights when your parents were gone and you were at home with a strange baby-sitter. It remembers the bad dreams and the terror you felt at waking up in the dark with repetitive nightmares. It will do anything to avoid repeating that pain!

That is why the Critic is generally such an enemy of the Inner Child. *For the Inner Critic, the vulnerability of the Inner Child and the feelings of pain, shame, and terror are irrevocably associated with one another.* The Critic must have us always in control, doing things right, feeling right, eating right, learning right, mothering right, working right. Then, maybe, we can be safe. If it had the power to do so, it would buy multiple antipain and antishame insurance policies to ensure our safety and well-being.

The Critic always sits on top of the Inner Child, keeping it down so that life will work right. The Inner Critic cannot come to us and say, "I'm feeling very vulnerable about the way you are eating. I'm afraid that you're going to become ill and not be able to work, and that is very frightening to me." That is the kind of thing that the Child might say to us. Instead, the Critic, always pushing away our vulnerability, says to us in its inimitably cold, rational, and judgmental tone, "You're such a slob. When will you ever have control? This stuff is poison for you. You're just weak."

When we apply the conversion principle to this statement and really go underneath the attack, we finally get to the vulnerability that lies at the heart of the Inner Critic. Then we hear its voice, sounding totally different, telling us how bad it feels about our eating and how frightened it is of illness and how confused it feels by all the conflicting information that is fed into it. We see that the Critic is really asking us for help because it feels so overwhelmed by the world and its demands and requirements. Then we find that as we learn to take care of the Critic we are also learning to care for the Inner Child.

JOURNAL WRITING

In the Voice Dialogue process, it is necessary to have a facilitator talk to your selves in order for you to become aware of these selves and learn to see, hear, and feel them. In addition, Voice Dialogue helps you to establish an Aware Ego by helping you become aware of and separate from your primary selves and ultimately become aware of and experience your disowned selves. Eventually, however, it is a good idea to learn how to address these selves on your own. One of the best ways of doing this is through journal writing.

Journal writing has been around for a long time. It was originally made popular by a Jungian-oriented therapist by the name of Ira Progoff. More recently, the journal process has been further developed and popularized by Lucia Capacchione, who has written a series of books on the subject. We recommend all of Lucia's books to you, though our emphasis would be on two of them: *The Power of Your Other Hand* and *Recovery of Your Inner Child*. In them she provides an in-depth discussion of journal writing, which we summarize here.

Journal writing is a natural process. After all, people have been writing in journals for hundreds, perhaps thousands, of years, and much of our information about the world and about historical figures is gained from personal journals. Traditionally, the writer writes about events, feelings, and ideas. What has been added to this process really began with the work of C. G. Jung and his process of active imagination. In this process, Jung began to carry on discussions with the figures of his inner world. He would write to dream figures, to inner voices, to sensations and feelings exactly as though he were carrying on a dialogue with another person, which in fact he was, though the person was on an inner rather than an outer level.

The process is very simple. You sit down in front of a notebook and begin to write from the "I" that is talking to one of the selves. It would look like this:

I: I wanted to talk to you because I've become aware of just how powerful you are and just how much influence you have in my life.

CRITIC (or any other self): Well, I'm glad that you appreciate just how important I am. If you would know that and always do what I say, things would go much better.

I: No, that isn't what I meant exactly. I appreciate your power, but I'm also becoming aware of how much on the muscle you are with me. You've been criticizing me all my life.

CRITIC: Well, better me than them. . . .

We can see how journal writing is a significant complement to Voice Dialogue. The more that we develop an Aware Ego that is separated from the different selves, the more effective is the "I" that talks to the different parts. Without any separation from these parts, it is not possible to engage in the dialogue process in journal work. What is important in this kind of writing is to put oneself into the writing as fully as possible. We need to involve our feelings and emotions as well as our minds. The more feeling we put into the dialogue, the more meaningful the outcome to us. Because of the simplicity and effectiveness of this process, it has become one of our main recommendations to people for continuing their explorations of their different selves.

Within us live all kinds of fascinating selves, in addition to the Inner Critic, that we can talk to in journal work. There is a Vulnerable Child, an Inner Therapist or simply an objective voice, a Supportive Parent, and a Wisdom Voice. We can speak to the Responsible Parent, Rebel, Shy Child, Magical Child, Pusher, Perfectionist, or Power Voices. There is no end to the possibilities for exploring the many selves that live within.

Sometimes people talk to the selves just in their own imagination, without writing them down in dialogue form. This too can be very effective; if it works, use it. Our experience, however, is that the writing tends to objectify the voices more clearly and strengthen the Aware Ego since it requires a stronger focus.

Other people describe allowing the voices to speak into a tape recorder, and yet others allow the different voices to sit in different places on couches and chairs in the living room. If we liken the selves to the varied musicians and instruments of an orchestra, then we must remember that it is the orchestra conductor who ultimately must be strengthened. It is the conductor who represents the Aware Ego, and without the conductor's power there is no way for all the disparate elements to be brought together in a way that can create lovely music. So whatever method you use to become aware of the different selves, please always keep in mind that the Aware Ego must remain the primary focus.

GETTING TO THE INNER CRITIC'S ANXIETY
THROUGH JOURNAL WRITING

John has begun to recognize the voice of his Critic. It is always criticizing his body. It tells him many things that are wrong with his body, but one of its primary criticisms is that he is losing his hair. It keeps telling him that he is becoming bald. John has spent much time scrutinizing his hair and trying to figure out how much it has changed. This has affected his relationships to women because he feels self-conscious and assumes that the woman is looking disapprovingly at his hair. Up until now, he has been the victim of his Inner Critic, which has functioned within him in much the same way his own mother functioned in his growing-up process. His mother was always scrutinizing him and commenting on what might be wrong with him.

Because of his Inner Critic work, John has learned to recognize station KRAZY. He has separated from his Critic. He has developed an Aware Ego that can hear its voice and that is beginning to have some choice about how to relate to it. One day he is writing in his journal, carrying on a conversation with the Critic. He asks the Critic, "Why are you always criticizing my hair? Why is this so important to you? It must bother you an awful lot. Why are you so upset?" He is no longer intimidated by the Critic. He is no longer fighting the Critic. He is quite impersonal about the whole thing and really wants to understand what is upsetting the Critic.

The answer of the Critic amazes John.

CRITIC (via the journal writing): I'm afraid that no one will ever want you and that you'll be all alone all your life.

JOHN: And why does that bother you so?

CRITIC: People won't respect you. They'll feel you can't get a woman. I'm afraid of all the judgments that people will make about you. And then too what will happen when you're old? I'm afraid of being alone with no one to take care of you.

John's dialogue with the Inner Critic continued. We have excerpted only a few sentences for illustration. How different this discussion from the years of attack and condemnation he had experienced! This time he has gotten beneath the Critic's attack rather than remain a worried victim to all its criticism. *He heard the attack as a call for help, and he went underneath to the fundamental issues of anxiety and vulnerability that have been fueling the Critic most of the years of his life.* No wonder so many people feel as though they have gotten out of prison when they make this discovery. Suddenly it is the Inner Critic that needs parenting rather than the other way around.

In contrast, Janet's Critic focused on her lack of organization. In Voice Dialogue sessions it would comment on how sloppy she was at work, how she never knew where anything was, and that it was a miracle that she was still able to survive on a job. Janet began to recognize the voice of the Critic, and she was beginning to sense its underlying anxiety. One day in the course of writing to her Critic, Janet asked it why it was always so upset about her lack of organization. She told it she was aware that she was not very well organized, but the Critic's concerns seemed much greater and deeper than this particular problem. The Critic answered her as follows:

CRITIC: It frightens me when you're not organized. Things feel out of control, and I'm afraid of what might happen.

JANET: What is it that you're afraid of?

CRITIC: Catastrophe! You might be fired. Someone might scream at you. I feel so terribly embarrassed when you misplace something because I'm afraid someone will find out and say something. Last week you couldn't find one of the files and I was terrified your boss would yell at you. He didn't, but it was a close call.

Janet has now applied the conversion principle to her Inner Critic. She hears the attack and she is aware that the Critic is frightened. Her vulnerability is threatened and the Critic is rising to its defense. Janet now has an Aware Ego in relationship to the Critic, so she is able to speak to it with compassion—no longer its victim, but at last able to bring to the Critic the support that it so desperately needs.

IN SUMMARY

As the Aware Ego develops through our readings and all of our psychospiritual work, it separates from the Inner Critic so that we are no longer identified with and victim to the Critic. We start listening to the Inner Critic with some objectivity. As this process continues, the attacking energy and voice of the Critic can be interpreted differently. We can see it as an alarm system that signals a call for help, a system that is alerting us to the possibility of pain, shame, and abandonment. It is as though the Inner Critic is dialing 911. "Emergency! Look out! Please help me because I cannot handle this situation!"

Thus the Inner Critic, because of our newly developed power and authority, takes on a different role. It, in essence, becomes a spokesperson for all of our vulnerability. When we have uncovered the underlying meaning of these attacks, it no longer hammers at us in the same way. We learn to handle the underlying problems about which it is concerned, and we learn to care for the Critic in a new way. How we care for the Critic is the subject of the next chapter.

Chapter Seventeen

Becoming a Parent to Your Inner Critic

When you learn to parent your Inner Critic you begin to assume control of the aspects of your life for which the Critic has until now been responsible. You assume the caring parental role in relation to the Critic. This is quite similar to taking responsibility for an elderly parent who has cared for you all your life and is no longer capable of performing this task but who, nonetheless, keeps on trying to parent you in the same old way. This parent now needs you to function independently and, in addition to this, desperately needs your help and support in dealing with the anxieties and problems of living although he or she does not know how to ask for this.

If you are identified with a primary self such as your mind, then that is who you think you are. In such a case, you live life primarily through your mind, and your feelings and emotions are fairly unimportant. There is no "I" to reflect on the fact that this is happening because your mind *is* the "I" of your life. Therefore, you have no choice in your actions, even though you believe that you do. It is your mind that determines your approach to life, work, and relationship.

If your primary self is a Responsible Parent, then you always take care of people and this is the "I" that you think you are. Without the knowledge that you are identified with a primary self, you would assume that you do have choice and are making conscious decisions about taking care of others. Once you become aware of the fact that you are identified with a self that always behaves responsibly, then you are in a position to separate from it. You are now able to become aware of the opposites within you. On the one side is your commitment to responsibility. On the other side is your commitment to taking care of yourself. Or on the one side is your mind with all of its power and authority and on the other side is your feeling reality. The idea is not to reject or judge your primary self. It is simply to understand that the primary self is not who you are so that you can begin to embrace both sides of yourself.

YOUR NEW ROLE IN THE PARENTING OF YOUR SELVES

You now have a new and very exciting job. The new "you," your Aware Ego, is born when you first begin to separate from your primary selves. Once this begins to happen, you can discover and experience the disowned selves on the other side. Once you know about the primary and disowned selves, you have the possibility of embracing the multiple opposites that live within you and learning to carry the tension of these opposites. Now you are ready for your new job, the extremely important job of assuming responsibility for your selves, of becoming parent to all the selves within you. When you do this, you have a new clarity of choice that was not previously available to you.

Every primary self, including the Inner Critic, was born to take care of you in some way. These selves are happy to give up the job once they feel that there is someone around who can run your life, and this someone, of course, is you. What does it mean for you to become parent to a self? Parenting a self means literally becoming the responsible agent for that self. *Since most of our primary selves, including the Inner Critic, develop in large measure to protect the Inner Child, none of these selves can relax and give up their control over our lives until we have taken full responsibility for the care of this Child and they are sure that we will meet its needs appropriately.* Therefore, let us first consider what it is like to take care of this Child.

When we talk to an Inner Child, it will often tell us exactly what it needs or likes or does not like. It is afraid of certain people. It likes to be with and feels safe with other people. It may be afraid of traveling. It may be afraid of groups of people. It may like to go for walks or take hot baths or have stuffed animals or watch cartoons on television. It may like to do nothing, just sit and stare with absolutely no requirements. Once we have identified the feelings of the child we are in a position to choose what needs to be done or not done. Parenting an Inner Child does not mean saying yes to all of its needs. It simply means that we remain related to the Child's needs, fears, and anxieties; that we treat it as a good parent should, comforting it and deferring to its needs and fears some of the time and encouraging it to be brave and take appropriate risks at others.

Let us say that your Inner Child is afraid of taking trips out of the country. This does not mean that you do not take trips. If we did not do any of the things that our inner children were afraid of doing, none of us would be doing very much. However, you might find out some of the things that would make your Child feel better. He or she might feel better if you had reservations to stay somewhere for the first few nights. Some children ask for their own pillows. Some like it when you take along extra food. Most of them like to know that they will be taken care of in an emergency—that there is enough money, medicine, and warm clothing. Many will ask that you bring along special books that they can enjoy. Others like you to write letters so that there is a feeling of being in touch with people back home. It is amazing how sometimes the smallest thing can make the Child feel better.

Parenting the Child means that we recognize the fear and anxiety and that we hear the pleas that the Child is making. Then we are in a position to make choices based on the overall situation. Whether you choose to do what the child wishes or not, the Child feels that it is being well cared for.

We remember an actress in one of our groups who frequently went on auditions for acting roles. She was terrified and often froze, losing many good roles. She gradually became aware of both her Critic and Child. Bit by bit, she discovered how terrified the Child was at these auditions and how the Critic's reactions were based on the terror felt by the Child. The client began to talk with the Child before her interviews. What could she do that would make the Child feel better? One of the things the Child asked for was a treat after the audition so she could look forward to something special. So the client began to plan special outings after the auditions—a special lunch or a visit to some special place or a special sweet or a special drive or activity that the Child wanted. The situation became quite manageable. It was not that the fear completely disappeared; it simply was that the call for help was heard and met. *It is not so much what we actually do or do not do; it is that we take the Inner Child or any other self seriously.* Each of our selves behaves like a real person and feels like a real person. Each needs our attention and needs to feel that it is being taken seriously. By taking care of her Child in this way, the actress became the responsible agent for her Child and the Critic became much less negative because it felt much safer.

Let us look at another example in which Susan learns to parent a primary self by learning to handle the Inner Child. Susan reached a point in her life where she separated from a primary self that was very responsible in its behavior toward people. Before this separation, she was the kind of person who was always available to her friends, for hours on end, with no consideration of her own needs. One day, after this new kind of understanding had come to her, the phone rang and it was one of her friends. She wanted very much to talk about some personal issues. The part of Susan that is mother to all of her friends immediately jumped in and was ready to listen for as long as necessary. Because of her new understanding, however, Susan knew that there was another side. She was able to tune in to a voice that represented the opposite side, and it told her something entirely different from what she had been used to hearing. It said to her, "This is not the time to talk. You have too much to do. Tell her you will call her back later."

Now Susan has some choice in this matter. She also has a conflict. The Inner Mother is terrified at the idea that Susan would tell her friend that she cannot talk to her, and Susan's Critic is having a full-scale anxiety attack. It accuses her of self-ishness. It tells her that no one will want her if she is no longer available to them whenever they need her. Nevertheless, her more selfish voice is sick and tired of always being available to everyone. How then can Susan parent both this Inner Mother and her Inner Critic in this situation?

The main way for Susan to parent both her more responsible self and the Critic is to feel their underlying vulnerability. Her maternal way of behaving in the world was born as a way of making Susan feel safe as a little girl. This internal mother is afraid of hurting her friend's feelings because this friend might abandon her if Susan is not available when needed and does not give to her. Also, this maternal self feels everyone's pain profoundly because it is so closely connected to the vulnerability and sensitivity of Susan. Therefore, it feels the pain of Susan's friends and makes sure that she gives to them, expecting that, in return, they will always be there for her and care for her. But Susan has noticed that this is not the way these relationships are actually working out.

Susan must now take over the parenting job and let the Inner Mother and the Critic know that they can relax, that it is not necessary to be available to everyone, that they have done a wonderful job but now she can take over and keep things safe. This means, however, that Susan must take over the job of protecting the Child. So long as it is left to the responsible self and the Inner Critic, Susan will be unable to establish any appropriate boundaries. An Aware Ego can say no if it chooses and can handle the anxiety that goes with establishing appropriate boundaries. *The parts of us that are always giving to people cannot maintain appropriate boundaries because they are terrified that we will be confronted, attacked, or abandoned by the people with whom we are dealing.*

AFFIRMATIONS

Affirmations are forms of meditation that are usually spoken or written. They are statements that are made to support the positive sides of a person, to help bring in healthier energy, and to draw in divine support. In addition to this, affirmations are one way of parenting the Inner Child and dealing with the negativity of the Inner Critic.

There are hundreds of affirmations, and the use of these as a meditation or as a reprogramming of the negative statements of the Critic can be very helpful and strengthening. Here are a few examples of affirmations:

God loves me.

I am divine.

I open my heart and love all those around me.

I am basically good and I close myself to negativity.

I am a channel for God's loving energy.

These affirmations are one way of dealing with the negativity of the Inner Critic as well as the negativity of one's actual life. As you can see, they are used to affirm the positive and healthy side of a person. The refrain of the Critic, "The trouble with you is . . ." is a kind of negative affirmation. Instead of affirming the individual, it is denying him or her.

Affirmations do not make the Inner Critic go away. Our basic experience is that one cannot get rid of negativity by trying to make things positive. Affirmations are really a way of developing a new, more positive self. The problem is that some Critics become stronger under these conditions, as though to balance the positiveness of the affirmation.

The ideal way to use affirmations, from our perspective, is to use them along with Inner Critic work, because a Critic ignored or directly challenged becomes an increasingly dangerous adversary. With this combination, you have the best of both worlds. You can take advantage of the tremendous support that affirmations can bring while at the same time learning to understand and handle the Inner Critic as we have described in this book.

PARENTING THE INNER CRITIC

In the beginning of this book, we took the first step toward dealing with the Inner Critic by learning to identify station KRAZY and to recognize when it was playing. Next we learned to listen to what it was saying—to identify the content that was being broadcast. Then we learned that it was possible to turn the station off or shift to a different station with better programming. Last, we learned that the attack of the Inner Critic, as played over and over on our mythical station KRAZY, is, in fact, an alarm. It is a call for help, and underneath its criticism is the Critic's fear, anxiety, and vulnerability about living in the world.

Now we have another step in the process. Now we begin to nurture the Inner Critic by starting to take over the functions that it has been handling. We have given a number of examples of how people become parents to the Inner Child and to certain of the primary selves. We did this so that you would better understand the concept of parenting your own Inner Family. Let us now examine what it is like to parent the Inner Critic directly.

Debbie is a very successful businesswoman, and she has had an equally successful Inner Critic accompanying her on her path to the top of her profession. Her Critic kept telling her that she really did not know what she was doing at work and that eventually someone was going to discover this and she would be finished. It also told her that she would never have a man because no man would be interested in her so long as she spent all her time on her career. In fact, she had quite a pleasant, albeit safe, social life, but as we know by now, Inner Critics do not exist to reward us for good behavior or for success. Debbie gradually became aware of the station KRAZY and its messages and began to have some choice about turning it off. She used journal dialogue to continue her direct contact with her Inner Critic and to deepen her awareness of its anxieties and needs.

DEBBIE: Why do you keep criticizing me about my job and about the fact that I'm never going to be married? What is it that really upsets you?

CRITIC: I'm very anxious about the job. You have so much responsibility. Men have that kind of responsibility, not women. I'm just terrified that you're going to make a fool of yourself and that no one will ever want to be with you.

DEBBIE: So you're feeling scared. That's what's behind all these years of criticism. That's what my mother used to say. She was terrified of the world, just like you are underneath. She also felt that it was a man's world.

CRITIC: Well, after years of listening to her, you can't blame me for feeling scared. You spent so much time trying to ignore her and learning to be strong and independent that you left me to carry all the anxiety. Well, I *am* afraid of the world. It scares me. And I would like to see us safe with a man who could take care of us. It frightens me to think of growing old all alone. How could a man ever want to be with you and have a family when you always act as though it doesn't really matter to you?

The Inner Critic is still making comments, but there is a totally different quality to the interaction. The Critic is now communicating from the feelings that have always been there underneath. The attack is over. Debbie can now listen to her Critic's ideas because she has successfully neutralized its negativity. She has gone beneath the attack to search for the vulnerability. Let us continue the dialogue.

DEBBIE: Look, I have to work. However, I also appreciate the fact that you're feeling very upset. What could I do for you that would make you feel better?

CRITIC: Stop working on Saturdays. Even if you work half a day, the day is shot. Stop trying to be a girl wonder. And begin to accept more dates. You act so independent. Take some risks and open yourself to some new men. Stop making me responsible for whether or not you get married. You know that you want to get married. I want you to feel what I'm feeling. Then I won't have to feel all these things for you.

DEBBIE: You know something? I'm going to consider these two things very carefully. I can't promise you at this moment that I'm going to do them, but I feel you have a real point. I'm beginning to see too that I haven't taken any responsibility for meeting men and even though I have a nice social life, it is a very safe one and it effectively keeps me from meeting new people. It's almost as though you have had to carry the anxiety about all this because I closed my eyes to it.

CRITIC: I always get the bad rap for these things. The Inner Child and I are terrified about being alone in the world and never having children and being all alone as you get older. I really would rather have you worry about it than me.

DEBBIE: Well, it really is my responsibility, not yours. I can't tell you that I'll be able to handle it all right away, but I really want you to have some time off. I think I'm beginning to understand what Jonathan (her therapist) meant when he said that you really needed a mommy to take care of you. I guess I'll be that mommy, once I'm able to handle the job. I'm going to start working on it right away.

Here we see the full transition from Debbie as victim of the Critic to Debbie as parent of her Critic. We see her recognizing the fears of the Critic and gradually beginning to assume the responsibility for dealing with these fears.

Like Debbie, when you learn to parent your Inner Critic you begin to assume control of the aspects of your life for which the Critic has until now been responsible. You assume the caring parental role in relation to it. This is quite similar to taking responsibility for an elderly parent who has cared for you all your life and is no longer capable of performing this task but who, nonetheless, keeps on trying to parent you in the same old way. This parent now needs you to function independently and, in addition to this, desperately needs your help and support in dealing with the anxieties and problems of living although he or she does not know how to ask for this.

As this shift of responsibility occurs, you can see how the negativity of the Inner Critic is neutralized and the Critic, using its special abilities to spot potential problems, becomes a part of your inner support system. The ideas of this Critic are now available to you as part of your objective mind and are directly and clearly related to the emotions and the needs of your Inner Child. Thus it is now an ally and no longer an adversary.

BECOMING MORE IMPERSONAL

You might note that when Debbie wrote to her Inner Critic in her journal, her tone (or energy) was *impersonal* rather than *personal*. She did not get upset, either when her Critic was negative or when it was worried. She listened carefully with some detachment. She did not try to make it happy. Instead she tried to figure out what was bothering it and what actions she might take. One of the best ways to deal with the Critic is to adopt this impersonal way of being in the world, both in relation to the Critic itself and to the outside world as well.

What do we mean when we speak of "impersonal energy"? When you are impersonal, you are not deeply concerned about your emotional connection to other people; you have well-defined boundaries, you are objective, and you are able to think and react clearly without being overly influenced by the feelings or reactions of others. This does not mean that you are withdrawn or angry; it just means that you, as an individual, are completely self-contained. What is your responsibility is yours, what is someone else's is theirs. You do not need them to feel or behave in any particular way.

"Personal energy," in contrast, means being hooked in to the feelings of others. When you live your life in personal energy, you feel a pressure to remain in emotional contact with others around you. If you feel them withdraw or sense their displeasure, you become upset. Your boundaries are not clearly defined so you are easily influenced by everything that is going on around you. Your strength in the world comes more from your relationship to feelings than your relationship to thinking. How other people feel in your presence or what they feel about you is of the utmost importance.

Just think of a classroom teacher. Lettie is a teacher who lives her life in personal energies. She is warm and absolutely charming, but she *must* have all her pupils like her. She cannot set limits or discipline effectively. She bounces back and forth between trying to entice her pupils into obedience and trying to frighten them into obedience by shouting at them. Even when she does an excellent job teaching, she finds that if one person gets upset with her it will ruin her day. Her Critic, ever anxious, is quick to point out all her mistakes and to review them over and over again. Every once in a while, life in the classroom gets so exhausting for Lettie that she feels she simply cannot go in another day and she withdraws completely. She has been putting out too much personal energy. Since she cannot set boundaries when anyone else is present, from time to time she just takes a day off, stays in her apartment, and reads. On these days she does not even answer the phone.

Linda, in contrast, is an excellent teacher who knows how to be impersonal in the classroom. She knows that if she needs to have all her pupils like her, she will be too vulnerable and will lose control of them. She will not be able to maintain order and the material that must be taught will not get covered. She is pleasant, fair, and objective, but she has a good sense of herself and her boundaries in this situation. She cannot be manipulated. Thus her Inner Child is protected, her vulnerability is not exposed to anyone, and her Inner Critic will not attack her.

Most women have been encouraged to be personal. Part of the patriarchal heritage is the idea that women should be warm, feeling creatures with endless compassion for humanity while men are expected to be cool, detached, and rational. Thus women are often actively discouraged during their growing-up years from being too objective, detached, or self-contained. It is simply seen as unfeminine.

When you live in personal energy, you tend to become a child to those around you. You are always vulnerable to their reactions. You can imagine the power that this personal way of living gives to your Inner Critic. It becomes your Critic's job to keep you in good emotional contact with those around you. It criticizes you if anyone is unhappy in your presence or withdrawn from you. Since you must feel close to others, your Inner Critic has a field day telling you all the things that are wrong with you that displease them.

Needless to say, when you adopt a more impersonal attitude, you have more distance and objectivity. Without becoming judgmental, you can see what is your part of an interpersonal difficulty and what belongs to the other person. When you are impersonal, you do not become desperate if others withdraw from you or judge you. You do not have to woo them back or to fight with them to reestablish some kind of emotional contact. Thus when you are impersonal and self-contained, you are less vulnerable to the whims of others. You are protecting your own vulnerability with adequate boundaries, and your Inner Critic has less need to be anxious. You are parenting it effectively by your reassuring ability to remain impersonal when necessary, thus avoiding some of the unnecessarily painful situations brought about by a more personal approach to life.

A SPIRITUAL ATTITUDE

A spiritual attitude or belief system can also help in parenting the Inner Critic. We are not talking here about a set of rules and regulations that require you to behave in a certain way. We are talking about a worldview in which you see yourself in relation to a greater whole, one that allows you to surrender to a higher power that supports you in the work of transformation.

When life becomes difficult, a spiritual attitude can be essential. It can give us a reason for living and a sense of meaning and purpose in life. This is often necessary before other kinds of psychological work can be done. There are in the world today an ever-increasing number of inspirational writers and teachers who help to initiate people into a spiritual approach to living and to spiritual states of consciousness. The entire Twelve-Step movement and the groups that follow its guidelines are built upon a spiritual foundation for transformation and growth. A multitude of books and tapes teach about spiritual awareness.

We have found that it can be particularly valuable to get in touch with an inner wisdom figure or a guide through Voice Dialogue, some form of journal writing, or the use of visual imagery. This kind of inner wisdom or spiritual voice can be very supportive and often provides a balance to the negativity of the Critic. It can help to deal with the Critic's underlying anxiety by providing information or suggestions that aid in the parenting process.

IF YOU NEED MORE

If you find that you have followed these suggestions and your Inner Critic is too powerful for you to deal with by yourself, please consult a counselor or psychotherapist. When you work with a therapist or a counselor, be sure that this feels right for you. Do not continue to see someone you do not like. Also remember that *therapy is not forever; personal growth is forever.*

You might also consider one of the many support groups that are available at this time. We have found that the Twelve-Step programs can be particularly helpful in giving support for dealing with both the Inner Critic and the shame that it engenders. Again, be sure that the group is appropriate and that you feel good about it.

Lastly, do not forget the possibility of antidepressant or antianxiety medications when these are properly prescribed and supervised by a physician. A number of new medications are extremely effective. Although we tend to emphasize the psychological aspects of depression and anxiety, we know individuals who have seen a lifetime of suffering come to an end with the administration of these drugs. Therefore, we would like to remind you that these are available and should most definitely be considered if you find that your psychological work alone is not adequate.

At the end of this book, we have included a list of recommended readings and audiotapes that we have found valuable in our own process of personal growth. The potential list is overwhelming, so we have included only those that have had particular meaning for us.

Chapter Eighteen

Moving Toward the Creative Life
The Inner Critic Transformed

When the negativity of the Inner Critic is finally neutralized, the ideas of the Inner Critic become an important part of your inner support system. They are now an aspect of your objective, discerning mind. The transformed Critic also helps to keep you safe. It gives you authority, objectivity, and the ability to set appropriate boundaries. This kind of support is like having a good internal parent who protects you and protects your creative process. In this way, you are freed to lead a creative life.

We are coming to the end of this particular journey together. It has been a pleasure for us to share with you the knowledge and experience we have gained from our many years of observing the Inner Critic—both our own and others'. As you may have noticed, the Inner Critic has been a never-ending source of amazement and fascination as well as a real challenge to us.

Our own attitude toward the Inner Critic has changed over the years. In the beginning, we treated the Critic as a wily and dangerous opponent. We tried to disempower it in whatever way we could. We joked about it, we played with it, we spent hours and hours exposing its cruelty and its contradictory demands, we exhorted people to do battle with it. Now we try to understand it. We look for its anxiety and ally ourselves with its underlying concerns rather than listen to its superficial complaints. Our aim is to help people to develop an Aware Ego that can assume responsibility for directly dealing with these concerns and can neutralize the destructive aspects of the Inner Critic as well.

What happens to the Inner Critic when the Aware Ego takes over this job of driving your psychological car? Just like in the fairy tales, it transforms. *When your Aware Ego assumes responsibility for your life and your Inner Critic no longer has to feel so anxious, it has a chance to use its many talents in a new, and fully supportive, fashion.* It actually develops within itself an awareness of your needs and takes these into consideration when it gives advice. It protects you and it protects your creativity. Those of you who are familiar with Jungian psychology may note some resemblance between the Inner Critic and the animus. In this particular transformation, the negative animus turns into a positive animus.

THE OBJECTIVE MIND

The Inner Critic has always had the ability to analyze—everything! Its intelligence is remarkable. As the Critic transforms, it retains this intelligence and the ability to analyze everything, but its analysis and evaluation no longer sound judgmental. It is now objective, and its observations are discerning rather than condemnatory. The key here is that you no longer feel dreadful when the Critic finishes its comments. You do not feel that you are always making mistakes or are beset by symptoms. You no longer fear that you have lost your last opportunity to succeed in life. The transformed Critic now looks at you, your life, and your work objectively and feeds you information about what it sees.

The Inner Critic now has the quality of a discerning, objective mind; you might even wish to rename it the Objective Mind. It is ultimately rational and will help you to think clearly and to make appropriate discernments. It can review a piece of work and, without judgment, point out what was good and what was not good. It can show you what is missing or where you might have done something differently. It can help us in editing this book. It will look over what we have written and suggest changes. It will not take us to task for being stupid or for making mistakes; it will merely show us how things could look better.

In a similar fashion, your Objective Mind can help you in whatever it is that you do. It tends to be quite impersonal. It can even take issues that are usually emotionally loaded and analyze them. It can deal with your looks: What are your better features and which ones do you wish to play down? It can help you immeasurably on your job or in your profession. It will review your reports, do a last-minute check on something that you have built or repaired, or evaluate what changes are needed in your department. If you are a therapist, it can point out that your last set of interventions did not work and perhaps you should try something else. In sports, it can monitor your performance and make suggestions that will help you to improve.

This transformed Critic can even assist you in your personal life. As your Objective Mind, it can help you to figure out your own motivations and to observe your own behavior and its effect on others. It can provide unbiased information to your Aware Ego about many aspects of your interpersonal relations, including dispassionate observations of the significant people in your life. It can help you in child rearing. It is invaluable in setting limits or protecting your own boundaries.

Just as the Inner Critic was able to operate in every arena of your life, so can its transformed counterpart, the Objective Mind. Its clear vision can help you make discernments whenever and wherever these are necessary.

FOCUS

Another gift that your transformed Critic can bring to you is the ability to focus your attention. Its perceptions are clearly focused rather than diffuse. Remember how it could concentrate on every detail? Now this ability can work in your favor. Instead of focusing on what is wrong with you, it can bring you this capacity to concentrate on even the smallest details in all areas of your life and work.

The Critic, because of its basically rational approach to life, is not distracted by feelings. Therefore it can maintain its focus despite distraction. With its ability to focus, the Critic brings patience. The Critic had unending patience in the past in its search for what was wrong, and it can now put that patience to work for you rather than against you.

DISCIPLINE

Your Critic's aim was to have you do your best so that you would be safe, loved, and successful in life. As an ally, your transformed Critic continues to pursue this goal. It will not settle for shoddy work or halfhearted attempts to deal with the challenges that life brings to you. If you try hard and do your best, it will be pleased; if not, it will continue to pressure you to do better.

However, this pressure is not the relentless, cruel pressure that it was previously. *As the Critic transforms, it becomes conscious of your limitations and vulnerabilities. Therefore, its demands will be reasonable.* There is one area in which its demands are particularly helpful. It admires, and insists upon, discipline. In this way, it acts like a good parent, helping you to achieve appropriate discipline in all aspects of your life.

AUTHORITY

Remember the unquestionable authority of the Inner Critic? We are talking here about the ring of authority that made all its pronouncements sound like absolute truth. When your Critic transforms, this authority is now available directly to you, giving you greater power in the world. This gift of the transformed Critic supports you in every aspect of your life. Your new authority enables you to present yourself without doubts and hesitations and to convey the impression that you know exactly who you are, what you think, and what you want.

You do not have to be a know-it-all or an objectionable bully. The authority is just there naturally. If you recall, it was never necessary for your Inner Critic to shout and threaten; it only had to whisper and you listened.

CONSCIENCE

A transformed Inner Critic has as its attributes not only objective thought, focus, discipline, and authority; it also has attributes that we have traditionally thought of as related to conscience. It is quite discriminating in its concern with questions of morality, of right and wrong.

In its negative state, the Critic often torments us with references to our basic "badness," sometimes suggesting that we are irrevocably flawed or unredeemably sinful. It seems as though we can never be good enough to please it. Even if our actions are worthy, the Critic can judge us on the evil of our thoughts or motivations. A transformed Inner Critic can objectively evaluate our actions in moral or ethical terms and thereby contribute valuable information to our decisions in life.

We each have a set of values and a sense of rightness and wrongness. Most of us would like to live up to certain moral standards, although we are not always clear as to what they are. We just do not feel good inside when we have gone against them. The transformed Critic can help us to clarify and then to live up to our own moral standards. It can bring to our attention the ways in which we might have behaved differently. Again, we do not mean that it berates us and makes us feel terrible about ourselves. It simply is straightforward and objective in its evaluation of our thoughts and actions. After all, at times we really need this help, especially from a supportive authority within.

FREEING YOUR CREATIVITY

Last, but certainly not least, you will notice that when your Critic is transformed your creativity is freed because the Inner Critic is no longer blocking it. You are in a position to listen to your own intuition and to allow your creative impulses to flow. You can live your life creatively and enjoy your own creative process.

We have always viewed the Inner Critic as a major interference to this creative process. How can any of us expect to live a creative life, to change, to come up with new ideas, or to take risks when the Inner Critic is telling us that nothing will ever work? How can we try to do something that nobody else has done when the Inner Critic is waiting to comment upon our mistakes? How can we finish a piece of work while the Critic is looking over our shoulders, showing us all the things that are wrong with it?

A powerful Inner Critic undermines our courage by pointing out our inadequacies and weakness. It terrorizes us. We freeze into mediocre imitation and cannot trust ourselves and our own creative process. *When the Critic is strong, the only safe way for us to be in the world is to be exactly like everyone else and never to try anything new or different.* This way it will not become anxious because it can find no faults in us.

Similarly, when the Critic is strong, it is almost impossible to engage in any creative or artistic activity. When we write, the Inner Critic has something negative to say almost before we can put the words on paper. It chokes us up so that we cannot sing or play instruments. Our painting or sculpting is subjected to its merciless and endless anxious critique. We become so self-conscious that almost nothing can move through us freely or with grace.

When the Inner Critic transforms as we have described, it can be used to support our creativity. It provides the focus, the form, and the discernment that is such an important part of shaping the creative process. It can provide the discipline that so often is necessary. We can listen to our intuition, create our own artistic products, and develop new ideas. Then the transformed Critic can help us look these over objectively and make the proper adjustments and corrections. It can also support us with its authority. It acts much like a good parent with an imaginative and creative child.

LIVING LIFE AS AN ENERGY DANCER

All is energy. Energy is neither good nor bad; it just is. The Inner Critic is an energy pattern that vibrates in a particular way. Each of the selves that we have spoken about is also a form of energy. Each vibrates in its own particular pattern. Each has a good side and a bad side.

You have seen how the energy pattern we call the Inner Critic can work against you, blocking everything that you try to do and making your life miserable until, in some instances, life almost does not seem worth living. You have followed with us, and together we have journeyed down the path of transformation. First you learned how to hear and to recognize your Inner Critic, then how to understand it, and finally, with your newly developed Aware Ego, you learned how to "dance" with it, not to master it. As a result of this, your Critic has begun to transform and the attributes that have been destructive can begin to be supportive.

Let us take this opportunity to remind you that this change is neither totally irreversible nor irrevocably permanent. *At times of increased stress and vulnerability, the Inner Critic has been known to revert to its old ways.* Please do not be discouraged. This is not a disaster nor is it a sign of failure; it is a completely natural occurrence. Just repeat the separation process. You know how to recognize your old pal, the Critic, and how to dance with its energies. Just remember that he or she has become frightened and is asking for help.

Using the Inner Critic as a teacher, we have shown you how to become aware of a self, or energy pattern, then how to separate from it, and finally how to dance with it. As with all energies, once you know about them, you are in a position to deal with them differently. They no longer need to take over and run your life. The gifts these selves bring you can be used and their negative aspects can be transformed, minimized, or avoided.

We began this book by welcoming you to the land of the Inner Critic. We end it by welcoming you to the land of the Aware Ego and to a new way of living in the world with your own natural creativity—as an Energy Dancer.

APPENDIX A

Rating Your Inner Critic

To be rated on a three-point scale of:

Rarely (1)   About Average (3)   Frequently (5)

Scores of 1–45—Small Inner Critic

Scores of 46–75—Medium-Sized Critic

Scores of 76–100—Very Strong Inner Critic

1. I wake up at night worried about the mistakes that I made the day before.

2. I replay conversations after I've had them to see what I've done wrong.

3. I don't like the way my clothes look on me.

4. When I'm with other people, I wonder if they're critical of me.

5. I'm cautious about trying anything new because I'm afraid of looking foolish.

6. I'm afraid people will laugh at me.

7. I worry about what other people think.

8. I often feel inferior to other people.

9. I wish I had a more attractive body.

10. When I look in the mirror, I check to see what's wrong with me.

11. When I read over something I've just written, I'm not satisfied with it.

12. I'm afraid that there's something basically wrong with me.

13. I wonder what other people would think of me if they really knew what I was like underneath.

14. I compare myself with other people.

15. I seem to attract judgmental people.

16. I question my decisions after I have made them and think that I might have done better.

17. When I say 'No' I feel guilty.

18. When I take a test like this, I'm sure that I don't do as well as other people.

19. I avoid taking risks if I can help it.

20. When I think about self-improvement I feel that there is something wrong with me that needs to be fixed.

TOTALS _____ _____ _____

TOTAL POINTS _____

APPENDIX B

The Top Twelve Traits of the Inner Critic

1. It constricts your ability to be creative.

2. It stops you from taking risks because it makes you fear failure.

3. It views your life as a series of mistakes waiting to happen.

4. It undermines your courage to change.

5. It compares you unfavorably with others and makes you feel "less than."

5. It is constantly warning you not to look foolish.

6. It is terrified of being shamed and so monitors all your behavior to avoid this.

7. It causes you to suffer from low self-esteem, and possibly depression, because it tells you that you are not good enough.

8. It can make looking at yourself in a mirror or shopping for clothes miserable because of its ability to create such a negative view of the body.

9. It can take all the fun out of life with its criticisms.

10. It makes self-improvement a compulsive chore because it bases the work on the premise that something is wrong with you.

11. It doesn't allow you to take in the good feelings that other people have toward you.

12. It makes you susceptible, and often victim, to the judgments of other people.

APPENDIX C

The Critic Transformed

The Top Ten Traits of Your Inner Critic as a Supporter

1. It acts like a positive parent who supports you, makes your risk taking safe, and allows you to be creative and flowing.

2. It is impersonal and does not allow you to worry about what others will think.

3. It helps you to set appropriate boundaries.

4. It is no longer interested in other people's criticisms, so they do not bother you. This helps to free you from the fear of shame or humiliation.

5. Its power gives you greater authority in the world.

6. It brings you the ability to focus clearly.

7. As an objective mind, it analyzes events and feelings coolly, without making either you or others wrong.

8. Its objective evaluations of situations help you to behave appropriately and with self-discipline.

9. It helps you to get appropriate consultation and advice without making you feel that this is a sign of inadequacy.

10. It can direct you to self-improvement as growth or as an adventure rather than as a chore because nothing is "wrong" with you. It does not talk about symptoms or problems.

APPENDIX D

A Brief Description of the Voice Dialogue Process

1. Two persons participate in the Voice Dialogue process. One is the facilitator and one is the subject.

2. The facilitator first establishes rapport with the subject and determines, together with the subject, what areas might be explored and what subpersonality they might start with.

3. When both are ready, the facilitator asks the subject to physically move to another chair or to move the existing chair to a new place in the room where the subpersonality is located. This is a subjective choice on the part of the subject.

4. The facilitator then begins a conversation with the subpersonality that can last from a few minutes to an hour or more. No attempt is made to judge or change the subpersonality that is being facilitated.

5. After the work is completed, the subject is asked to return to the place where he or she was originally sitting. From this place a discussion occurs about what has been done.

6. As part of this discussion, the subject is asked to stand in the position of awareness while the facilitator summarizes the work that has been done.

7. It is possible for the facilitator to move the subject to another subpersonality and hence another seat before returning to the original position. Or, having done the summary, it is possible for the facilitator to continue the work by talking to a different subpersonality.

8. The determination of which selves to work with, when to work with opposite energies, how many selves to work with,

and how deeply to take the subject is a function of the training and experience of the facilitator. Voice Dialogue is not a parlor game and should not be used without appropriate training.

9. In the course of this work, no attempt is made to judge or change a self that is being facilitated. Also, the facilitator does not have the different selves talk to each other. We do not try to have the selves reconcile their differences with each other. Rather, our aim is to develop an awareness of them and to develop an Aware Ego that can embrace them in their uniqueness and their totality, no matter how different or opposite they may be.

10. The Voice Dialogue process can be used in relationship to any therapeutic system. What determines its power and its difference from other ways of working is the ability of the facilitator to "hold the energy" of the part being worked with. This requires focus and concentration. It also requires that the facilitator must have experienced in himself or herself the part that is being facilitated. This is what gives the subject the feeling of the total reality of each self.

11. A full discussion of Voice Dialogue can be found in *Embracing Our Selves,* which is listed in the bibliography. A somewhat longer description than this one can be found in chapter 2 of this book.

APPENDIX E

In a More Humorous Vein

Our Fantasies About the Top Eight Industrial Benefits of the Inner Critic

1. It is a major support of the psychotherapy industry.
2. It helps support the plastic surgery industry.
3. It helps support the self-help movement.
4. It strongly supports the sale of New Age books.
5. It supports the sale of cosmetics.
6. It solidly supports judgmental people in the world and helps them to prosper in their judgments.
7. It supports the sale of over-the-counter medications such as aspirin.
8. It helps to maintain the sale of alcohol and drugs.

RESOURCES

Books and Tapes

Bradshaw, John. *Healing the Shame That Binds You*. Deerfield Beach, FL: Health Communications, 1988.
———. *Homecoming*. New York: Bantam Books, 1992.
Capacchione, Lucia. *The Power of Your Other Hand*. Van Nuys, CA: Newcastle Publishing, 1988.
———. *The Recovery of Your Inner Child*. New York: Simon and Schuster, 1991.
Conger, Carolyn. *The Sacred Pool*. Audiotape. 1991. Available from Conger Seminars, P.O. Box 1447, Apple Valley, CA 92307.
———. *Vision Quest*. Audiotape. 1991. Available from Conger Seminars, P.O. Box 1447, Apple Valley, CA 92307.
Gawain, Shakti. *Creative Visualization*. San Rafael, CA: New World Library, 1978.
———. *Living in the Light*. San Rafael, CA: New World Library, 1986.
———. *Return to the Garden*. San Rafael, CA: New World Library, 1989.
Hesse, Hermann. *Steppenwolf*. New York: Henry Holt & Co., 1927.
Jung, C. G. *Memories, Dreams, Reflections*. Ed. A. Jaffe. New York: Pantheon Books, 1963.
Kazantzakis, Nikos. *The Odyssey: A Modern Sequel*. New York: Simon and Schuster, 1958.
Medicine Eagle, Brooke. *Buffalo Woman Comes Singing*. New York: Ballantine, 1991.

Stamboliev, Robert. *The Energetics of Voice Dialogue*. Mendocino, CA: LifeRhythmn Publishing, 1992.

Stone, Merlin. *When God Was a Woman*. New York: Dial Press, 1976.

Taegel, William. *The Many Colored Buffalo*. Norwood, NJ: Ablex Publishing, 1990.

The Mendocino Series
Audio Cassette Tapes by Hal Stone and Sidra Stone

THE PSYCHOLOGY OF SELVES: GROUP 1

Meeting Your Selves: An Introduction to the Psychology of Selves
This introductory tape teaches how to recognize and understand the amazing family of selves that lives within each of us. It explores how they develop and how they influence our lives. This is a wonderful beginning to the study of "The Psychology of Selves."

The Child Within
Within each of us lives an Inner Child who carries our essential being and who embodies our sensitivity to the world around us. It is this self that our other selves develop to protect. In this tape, you will be introduced to this Child. You will hear it speak and will learn how to listen for the almost inaudible voice of your own Child.

Meet Your Inner Critic
Everybody has an Inner Critic who is an authority on everything. It is the part of us that always has something critical to say. It is brilliant and perceptive, and when it whispers in our ears it usually sounds absolutely accurate in its uncharitable view of us, our behavior, and our achievements. Learn how to separate from yours!

Meet Your Inner Critic II
Further adventures with the Inner Critic. Hear it speak and gain greater understanding of its power in your life. Even if you

know about your Inner Critic already, we suggest that you listen to "Meet Your Inner Critic" first.

THE PSYCHOLOGY OF SELVES: GROUP 2

Meet the Pusher
The Inner Pusher is a driving force in our lives. This is the self that creates your agenda, tells you what you should do, accomplish, finish, read, write, create, etc. It can accomplish much, but it can also keep you in a constant state of dissatisfaction and can even erode your health. Learn how this Pusher operates in your life.

Integrating the Daemonic: Our Lost Instinctual Heritage
There is darkness and there is light! We cannot banish the darkness, but we *can* bring in the light. In this tape, Hal and Sidra focus the light of consciousness on the "darker" side of our human nature, showing how our disowned instinctual energies become daemonic and how we can reclaim these energies and bring them into our lives in a constructive fashion.

The Dance of the Selves in Relationship
"Each relationship brings with it the possibility of never-ending fascination and growth, but it also carries within it the seeds of its own destruction." Building upon the ideas introduced in "Meeting Your Selves," this tape introduces Hal and Sidra's revolutionary no-fault approach to relationship. It explains how you can make each of your relationships an exciting and positive experience, using relationship itself as a teacher, a healer, and a guide.

Understanding Your Relationships
This tape is a continuation and a deepening of the ideas presented in "The Dance of the Selves in Relationship." It will teach you how to decode the message of your relationships—how to analyze them and how to make sense of the confusion and discomforts of relational issues—because each of your relationships is a teacher if you understand the message that it brings to you.

VOICE DIALOGUE TRAINING TAPES: GROUP 3

Introducing Voice Dialogue
This is a step-by-step introduction to the use of Voice Dialogue, an incomparable tool for contacting the many selves. It provides a basic understanding of the Voice Dialogue process and its many uses.

Voice Dialogue Demonstrations
This is a teaching tape. Through the dramatization of Voice Dialogue sessions, you, the listener, can gain a firsthand experience of the process as it would be used in actual facilitation.

THE DREAM PROCESS: GROUP 4

Decoding Your Dreams
This tape is a treasure for anyone wishing to understand the language of dreams. It is a general guide for making sense of your dreams—those magical messages from the deepest parts of yourself, which can provide you with amazingly accurate practical information as well as profound spiritual teachings. Hal Stone's Jungian background gives an added depth to the lifetime of experience with dreams that is summarized and clearly presented by both Hal and Sidra on this tape.

Exploring the Daemonic in Dreams
The unconscious has its own special way of calling attention to the "daemonic" aspects of our psyches—the natural instinctual energies that we have disowned over time. These dreams, drawn from a number of countries, are remarkable for their clarity and intensity. They give a picture of the disowning process itself and of the importance of reclaiming our lost instinctual heritage.

Audiotapes, books, and information regarding training activities of Hal Stone and Sidra Stone are available from:
Delos, Inc.
P.O. Box 604
Albion, California 95410